WM400.P

D1253354

ELECTRICAL AND DRUG TREATMENTS IN PSYCHIATRY

Electrical and Drug Treatments in Psychiatry

by

A. SPENCER PATERSON

M. A. (Oxon.), M. D. (Edin.), F. R. C. P. (Edin.), M. R. C. P. (Lond.)

Senior Consultant Psychiatrist, West London Hospital (Charing Cross Group)

Consultant Psychiatrist to the French Hospital, London

ELSEVIER PUBLISHING COMPANY

AMSTERDAM — LONDON — NEW YORK

1963

SOLE DISTRIBUTORS FOR THE UNITED STATES AND CANADA

AMERICAN ELSEVIER PUBLISHING COMPANY, INC.

52 VANDERBILT AVENUE, NEW YORK 17, N.Y.

SOLE DISTRIBUTORS FOR GREAT BRITAIN

ELSEVIER PUBLISHING COMPANY LIMITED

12B, RIPPLESIDE COMMERCIAL ESTATE

RIPPLE ROAD, BARKING, ESSEX

LIBRARY OF CONGRESS CATALOG CARD NUMBER 62-19697

WITH 9 ILLUSTRATIONS AND 4 TABLES

Preface

When a book on a psychiatric subject was required for this series, I suggested that one on electrical and drug treatments would be suitable. These are the two physical therapies which are most widely employed at the present time in psychiatry and yet there is remarkably little information given about them in the textbooks. In other branches of medicine the clinician does not treat the patient until he understands the pathology of the disease and the pharmacological action of his remedy. In psychiatry however the exact mode of action of these compounds is more obscure and the writers of some textbooks have simply referred to both therapies as empirical, thus implying that nothing is really known about them. This however is very far from being the case. In this book an attempt is made to give the requisite information that is lacking in most textbooks.

There has in fact been a renewed interest in electrical treatment in the last two years. Its value in schizophrenia, which was put in doubt by some authorities, has now been accepted. While in the past junior doctors in mental hospitals have been advised to use the simplest possible machine and avoid premedication with muscular relaxants, nowadays they are officially advised to work with an anaesthetist. The latter is apt to take a different view of electrocerebral treatment from that held by the psychiatrist of ten years ago. The psychiatrist and anaesthetist now question whether an epileptic fit with a crude machine is the last word in electrocerebral treatment. The fit represents a maximum excitation of the nervous system but one wants to know about the possibilities of electrical inhibition, electric coma, electrically induced mental dissociation and abreaction, electrical anaesthesia and electrical sleep. Such treatments have certain advantages over the administration of pharmaceuticals. Electrical treatments are quick in obtaining results. They often make psychotherapy and rehabilitation possible early in the illness. They are humane and they have almost no side-effects. When the main course of treatment is completed it is seldom necessary to continue with maintenance therapy.

Part I of this book consists of an account of electrocerebral treatment.

As in the case of electric treatment, textbooks have not kept pace with the development of psychotropic drugs. These have been very successful in certain types of illness. They have been used either alone or in combination with electrical treatment.

Part II gives some account of the more important psychotropic drugs employed in the treatment of schizophrenia, the manic-depressive psychoses, and in the neuroses. In addition to the information given in the main text there is an appendix which can be pulled out and unfolded. In this way it is possible to see at a glance the main items such as generic and trade names, chemical structure, dosage, indications etc. and to refer them to the material in the main text. One can also easily compare the effects of one drug with those of another. At the present time there is no book to our knowledge which includes such a chart.

This book is based on work carried out at the Psychiatric Department of the West London Hospital during the past seventeen years. During the 1940's we realised that the stress treatments applied to patients suffering from early functional psychoses was the most important development in psychiatry since the advent of systematic psychotherapy in the neuroses. In 1947 we formed a team consisting of an anaesthetist, a physicist, a neurophysiologist and psychiatrist to study these problems.

Since 1950 we have had a neurophysiological laboratory with a full-time physiologist and have studied the different types of electrocerebral treatment mentioned above. Since 1959 we have also had a conditioned reflex set-up in which we have studied among other subjects the pharmacology of some psychotropic drugs.

The department has a dozen psychiatrists on the staff so that our clinical material has been extensive.

This book is intended both for psychiatrists and for general practitioners. Nowadays practitioners have been deprived of much of the work which was carried out by their predecessors, such as surgery, midwifery or the treatment of infectious diseases. However the community is relying on them to carry out a considerable amount of psychiatric treatment They see psychiatric emergencies and they have patients who have been discharged from a mental hospital entrusted to them for supervision and drug treatment. They are also learning the best drugs with which to treat neurotic patients. In addition, practitioners in other specialties, especially neurology and public health, are acquiring a new interest in psychiatric treatment.

I am particularly indebted to the Dan Mason Foundation for repeated grants which have enabled our investigations to be continued.

I am indebted to Professor T. Gualtierotti, who is now head of the Istituto di fisiologia umana, University of Milan, for his collaboration with me for three years at the West London Hospital and for recommending three of his pupils, Drs. Spinelli, Passerini and Bracchi to succeed him there.

On the clinical side I have received a great deal of help from my colleagues Drs. Felix Brown, Glyn Davies, Denis King, J. Runes, L. Field, B. Cwynar, and J. T. Robinson. The last-named has given me the benefit of his experiences with "LSD" treatment at Roffey Park which in described in Part II.

I am grateful to the following for help in preparing the book: Dr. J. Runes for reading the text, and Dr. J. Frisch for advice regarding pharmacology.

Finally, I am grateful to Mr. A. G. Stevens of the Malven Electrical Co., 284 London Road, St. Albans, for constructing instruments to meet some of our particular needs.

London, July 1962   *A. Spencer Paterson*

Contents

Part I, Electrical Treatment

Part II. Drug Treatments

PART I

Electrical Treatment

Introduction

The discoveries in the 1930's, of the administration of insulin comas (Sakel, 1936), of convulsive therapy with cardiazol (Meduna, 1937), and of electroshock (Cerletti and Bini, 1938), for the treatment of the functional psychoses, together marked the beginning of a new era in psychiatry. During the subsequent 20 years the success of these therapies caused a revolution in the mental health services of countries all over the world. In the 1950's several reports appeared in which treatment in the early 1930's was compared with that in mental hospitals 20 years later. Cook in his Presidential Address to the Royal Medico-Psychological Association (1958) described the state of affairs at Bexley Hospital near London in June 1935, when he took over charge of the female side. Most of the hospital was occupied by chronic patients. Out of 18 wards only 2 had open doors. There were 2 wards of some 70 patients, each composed mainly of chronic melancholics who had been in hospital from 2 to over 20 years. Although they had lost the acute edge of their depression they were preoccupied with delusions of unworthiness, hopelessness and bodily illness. Even larger numbers of chronic schizophrenics with far less prospect of remission occupied the other wards. These could be divided into 3 roughly equal groups: *(i)* Those whose psychosis was, so to speak, "burnt-out", and who were occupied more or less in automatic routine work; *(ii)* those who had sunk into a state of apathy and emotional dilapidation, and *(iii)* those who showed phases of excitement and violence, with noisy, turbulent and destructive behaviour. In the refactory wards there was a sustained atmosphere of tension; struggles and minor casualties were numerous. The chief medication consisted of giving paraldehyde and chloral hydrate, and 1,430 lbs of the former and 273 lbs of the latter were doled out annually ($=$ 648.5 and 124 kg respectively).

Cook comments: "In general I do not think that it is an overstatement to say that physical treatments have provided our most effective means of rendering the bulk of chronic patients more accessible to social rehabilitation or that the change of atmosphere of the chronic wards, which I have just described, must be attributed primarily to such procedures as convulsion therapy, leucotomy, and more recently tranquillizing drugs."

He then described the effects produced by the administration of ECT. "First of all it has proved a great boon in the case of endogenous depressions and in other such states as severe mania, acute puerperal psychoses, severe toxic confusional states and some fulminating schizophrenic reactions, occasionally preventing death from suicide or exhaustion. Secondly it has exerted a considerable influence on the morale of prospective patients and of their relatives and in fact upon the general public. It has not only proved time and again to be dramatically successful in severe and most alarming mental illnesses, but has altered the apparently hopeless course of thousands of long-standing psychoses, both schizophrenic and depressive. Without convulsion treatment the bed problem in mental hospitals might well by now have become insuperable." The writer goes on to state that convulsive treatment has been a basic factor in making possible the subsequent sweeping administrative changes in local mental health services throughout the country.

An article emanating from the same mental hospital (Norton, 1961) describes the female side in the year 1960. By that year the number of female beds had fallen from 1284 (in 1954) tot 1165, that is, a decrease of 119. This was parallel to what had been happening elsewhere, for in England between 1956 and 1959 there had been a drop in the number of beds to the extent of 15,000, a peak having been reached in 1954 of 148,600. Despite this fall in the number of beds, in the country as a whole there has been an increase in the number of new patients of about 125 per cent since 1946 (Paterson, 1959).

Norton had had the clinical impression that far fewer patients were becoming chronic and he therefore carried out an exhaustive investigation from April 1957 until January 1960. He compared the progress of patients during this period with that of patients who were admitted at intervals during the previous 30 years. In his hospital ECT was the treatment most used for schizophrenia until 1957. Only then did the administration of chlorpromazine become important. Insulin coma treatment was not very much used. The average age of the schizophrenics on admission was higher in the later period and this is probably explained by the fact that the younger schizophrenics were being treated at clinics on an ambulatory basis or in general hospitals, where there was a psychiatric service. The median stay in hospital for a schizophrenic was only 9 weeks instead of the 7 months during an earlier period 1928-30. Only 19 per cent of schizophrenics were still in hospital after 2 years instead of an average of 40 per cent in 1928-30. In 1957, 86.7 per cent of the patients admitted with schizophrenia were out of hospital within a year compared to 26.5 per cent 30 years previously. The duration of stay for a schizophrenic nowadays is not much greater than that of patients with an affective psychosis. By the end of two years only 10 per cent of schizophrenic admissions were still in hospital compared to 59 per cent 30 years previously. The proportion of schizophrenics in hospital 6 years after their admission in 1953 was only 12 per cent but at the end of 5 years beginning in 1928, 35 per cent were still in hospital.

Norton considers that a variety of factors has contributed to this remarkable outcome. First may be put the efficacy of the physical treatments, secondly the changed atmosphere of the hospital and thirdly a readiness on the part of relatives and the community to accept improved patients at home without too much apprehension. He remarks that those improved patients who leave hospital may have to return if circumstances become difficult at home, but these readmissions are merely episodes in the long term management of a patient who, had he become ill 30 years ago, would have had only 2 chances in 5 of ever being discharged.

With regard to the manic-depressive psychosis the length of stay in hospital has fallen from 6 months to 7 weeks and the proportion of those who leave hospital within a year has improved from 50 per cent to 90 per cent. The major part of this change occurred before 1949, that is to say before there were any administrative changes in the hospitals. Hence the most probable explanation of the improved outlook and shortened stay is the success of ECT. By 1949-50, 55 per cent of admissions for manic-depressive insanity were recovering with ECT and in 1957, 81 per cent were responding well to ECT, but of these 24 per cent needed more than a single course.

Such has been the success of ECT in schizophrenia according to Norton that recently organic dementia has taken the place of the latter as the commonest cause of stay in Bexley Hospital for more than 2 years. In

England nearly half the beds in the National Health Service were occupied by mental hospital patients and schizophrenia was the illness from which most of these long-stay patients suffered. That it is no longer the chief cause of the occupation of long-stay beds marks a turning-point in the history of psychiatry.

Another relevant study is that of a Scandinavian psychiatrist Achte (1961) from a mental hospital in Helsinki. He compared the biennium 1930-32 with 1952-54. The figures which he quotes are comparable with those reported by Norton. He says that shock treatments have abolished the feeling of hopelessness towards mental disorders which was prevalent in the public mind. Patients have ceased to be suspicious of psychiatrists and now co-operate with them. Their attitude to the psychiatrist has become more like that which they show towards their family doctor. For this reason patients come earlier to hospital.

This change in the attitude of patients and public alike was one of the most striking features of the era following the advent of shock treatments and electrical treatments in particular. In Buckinghamshire for example, the area served by the hospital which forms the subject of Shepherd's (1957) well-known monograph, members of the public were saying between 1939 and 1943 when shock treatments were given on a big scale, that doctors had found a cure for insanity, and so patients came willingly to have treatment.

A similar changed atmosphere prevailed at Portsmouth where T. Beaton, in 1945, had created a mental health service whereby patients could be seen early at the psychiatric clinic of a general hospital. It certainly appears that one of the major factors in the complete change in the attitude of the public to insanity was the widespread use of convulsive therapy in Portsmouth at that time. The government-sponsored report on the Mental Health Services written by C. P. Blacker (1946) refers to the situation in Portsmouth in 1945. He mentions that one of the methods used by Beaton to ensure that psychotic patients were treated early was to give demonstrations to local doctors of the effects of ECT on the psychoses.

The discovery in the 1950's of the phenothiazines and also of antidepressive drugs led to further success in the treatment of patients by physical methods: the initiation of the National Health Service in 1948 enabled those suffering from mental and nervous disorders to benefit to the maximal extent from these new developments. It is estimated that in Great Britain 90 per cent the psychiatric patients are actually treated compared with only 10 per cent in some other Western countries.

Hopeful as these trends are however, they certainly give no grounds for complacency; as the late Vera Norris (1959) said, in her monograph dealing with mental illness in London, "the prognosis for schizophrenia is still gloomy. About one third of the persons admitted to mental hospitals are not likely to recover sufficiently to leave hospital permanently; the chance of a person recovering sufficiently to leave hospital even after three years' continuous hospital care is small. Of those patients who recover enough to leave the mental hospital, over one third will be admitted at least once again within the ensuing four years ... There is reason to believe however that the prognosis is less gloomy (in 1954) than fifteen years or more ago, since the outcome for the unselected schizophrenics included in this study was almost as good as that for a group specially selected in 1933-34 for its favourable prognosis." Of manic-depressive psychosis Norris has this to say: "... of 100 persons admitted with this diagnosis about 50 will spend more than 16 weeks continuously in hospital and 9 will spend at least 4½ years continuously in hospital. The average expectation of stay in hospital is just under one year. Of 100 discharges, 40 are likely to be readmitted once, and of these 20 do have at least two readmissions within about 4 years of discharge." Norris sums up: "Optimism about the value of new methods of treatment should not lead to neglect or understatement of the enormous public health problem set by the two major psychoses, schizophrenia and manic-depressive psychosis."

This is a salutary warning against over-optimism, but there are three important ways in which genuine changes do appear to have occurred. First, many patients who have the most favourable prognosis are now being treated on an outpatient basis at general hospitals, and therefore do not become included in statistics of mental hospital admissions; secondly patients who previously may have become a part of the chronic mental hospital population are able to spend longer periods in the outside world, even though they may have to be readmitted from time to time for acute episodes. "The open door may become the revolving door." Thirdly, there can be little doubt that physical treatments have made possible the changes in the social rehabilitation within the hospital itself. Fig. 1 from Freyhan (1961) indicates that there has been a steady increase since 1908

References p. 100

in the number of patients able to return home from a typical mental hospital within the first 3 years of stay.

The work of Carse (1959) in which he shows how patients can be treated at an early stage without entering a mental hospital has depended largely on ECT. The success of physical treatments is greatly magnified by the efficient organisation for mental health in Great Britain. This gives scope for energetic psychiatrists at the periphery to work out an efficient local service: mention may be made for instance of Bowen and Crane's (1958) report from York and MacMillan's from Nottingham (1956). In fact some five hundred outpatient departments have been started in the past two or three decades, especially in the teaching hospitals and many of these have been started in the past ten years (see also Brown *et al.*, 1961; Mc Walter *et al.*, 1961; Morissey and Sainsbury, 1959; Royal Commission, 1957).

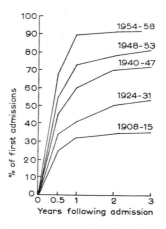

Fig. 1. Schizophrenia. Initial separation rates for first admission: comparison of selected cohorts, 1908-58 (F. A. Freyhan, in: E. Rothlin (Ed.), *Neuro-Psychopharmacology*, Vol. 2, Elsevier, Amsterdam, 1961, p. 192).

At the West London Hospital Psychiatric Clinic the number of patient sessions since 1945 has increased five times and the number of psychiatrists from 3 to 10 (Paterson, 1959). The need then arose for a neurophysiological laboratory. We have studied particularly problems connected with electrocerebral treatment since 1945 with a view to diminishing as far as possible the dangers and unpleasant side-effects, while at the same time attempting to increase its therapeutic efficiency to the maximum. In the 1940's we formed a team consisting of a psychiatrist, a physician, a neurophysiologist, an anaesthetist and a physicist. Incidentally we published a film in 1947 showing what are considered the best techniques for giving ECT. The technique of ECT described by us, though not wholly original, was little used at that time but has since become the standard method, except for the substitution of suxamethonium for curare. This short-acting relaxant which we first used in February 1952 has constituted the biggest single improvement in technique since the inception of ECT. It has made it easier to give concentrated ECT and so electronarcosis has come to be less used.

In the 1940's we realised that ECT was not specific for depression. It was merely that depression in general required fewer treatments than most other psychotic conditions including schizophrenia. On the Continent Cerletti (1950), Lopez Ibor (1950) and others recognised the nonspecificity of ECT and obtained excellent results in a variety of conditions, as will be reported later. It remained true however that the most carefully compiled statistics on schizophrenia showed rather better results with insulin coma treatment than with convulsion treatment. For this reason the University clinics in England advocated insulin coma as specific for schizophrenia. It was not appreciated that as patients came to be treated at a much earlier stage in their illness, ECT was sufficient to cause a lasting remission in most types of cases.

Progress in the study of electrocerebral treatments however during these years has been difficult because of a number of prejudices and mistaken ideas, many of which have been particularly prevalent in England. The following are some of these.

(i) That "as psychotic illness is caused by psychological conflict, it must be cured by psychotherapy". It is said that physical treatment only *appears* to help the patient and this appearance is because of injury done to the brain. The answer to this is that psychotherapy is suited for the neuroses but even as Freud said, it is not primarily indicated in the functional psychoses; there are affected by physical treatments in such a way that psychotherapy can ultimately take effect. Even at the Menninger Clinic ECT is employed.

(ii) That it is immoral to use ECT, as it is an insult to the patient and his dignity as a human being. Some such opinion was held by the French psychiatrist Baruk but even he has recently been using electroshock.

(iii) Some neurologists have criticised psychiatrists for using electroshock because it might injure the brain but it has been shown that there are almost no irreversible effects produced by the treatment. This was shown especially by Globus *et al.* (1943) in the case of electronarcosis, and they were found to be relatively slight in the case of ECT (Hartelius, 1952).

(iv) It was said that ECT was specific for depression, especially retarded depression, and that depressions had a non-reactive phase at the beginning when ECT should not be given. It is even said that one should wait till the patient is on the mend and then he should be given one a week. This is quite contrary to our experience. If a patient is given treatment at the beginning and if it is given in sufficient quantity, then a favourable result can be expected and a recurrent depression, which could last 3 months, lasts only 14 days. In the case of agitated melancholia however it is often advisable to give two treatments on the first day, to repeat this if necessary on the second day and to give treatments on successive days at the beginning of the illness. Nowadays when one can add such drugs as librium and tofranil, the prognosis is still better. If the opinions cited above of ECT were correct, then it would not be worth giving it at all, because the patient would already be recovering from a self-limited disease.

(v) That "if ECT cures depression, it is likely to be bad for other syndromes like mania or anxiety state". This belief arose from a failure to recognise that ECT was a non-specific treatment. One of the earliest discoveries Cerletti (1950), Lapipe and Rondepierre (1942) and Lopez Ibor (1950) made was that if ECT's were given with a larger number of treatments many other conditions such as mania and schizophrenia responded equally well. It was eventually found that what was important was that treatment should be given early. Although electroshocks given in small amounts make anxiety states worse, there is no doubt that concentrated ECT or electronarcosis can have a great success in the treatment of severe chronic anxiety.

(vi) That "concentrated ECT causes incurable dementia in many patients". There has been in England a great deal of confusion regarding the definition of concentrated ECT. In some countries chronic schizo-

phrenics have been treated with concentrated ECT to the extent of becoming doubly incontinent. Such treatment however is not much used now because it is known that the successful treatment of schizophrenia by ECT depends on the number of treatments given and not on giving it in a concentrated form.

(vii) That "the use of pentothal and muscle relaxants is more dangerous than giving ECT straight". It has been said that the giving of an anaesthetic and a relaxant "adds two more dangers to the patient". This view is no longer held because their use has practically eliminated dangerous side-effects from the treatment.

(viii) That "it is quite satisfactory for ECT to be given by the most junior Registrar without the help of an anaesthetist and without even having been trained by an anaesthetist". This fault has been the result of many authoritative psychiatrists not paying sufficient attention to the importance of this subject. In many hospitals now it is routine for an anaesthetist to help with the treatment. Where this does not pertain, then the worker ought to be seconded to another hospital where he can learn the treatment thoroughly and obtain a diploma in anaesthetics just as general practitioners can do.

(ix) That "the success of ECT shows that mental disorder is entirely of physical origin and that therefore psychotherapy and rehabilitation are unimportant". This is certainly not our experience and some of our most successful psychotherapy has been carried out on patients who have had electrocerebral treatment.

(x) That "ECT can be ignored as it is on the way out". It is true that in the years following 1952, ECT came to be used to a lesser extent (see Perr, 1961; Pichot, 1960). The advent of imipramine and other antidepressive drugs also led to a further decrease in its use. At the West London Hospital for a time we had almost given up the use of ECT. However we came to recognise that there were some patients who did not recover unless they were given this treatment. The anti-depressive drugs though valuable in many cases have not confirmed the high hopes which attended their introduction. We are once again using ECT and other forms of electrical therapy almost as much as in the past.

References p. 100

CHAPTER 1

The Pathology of the Functional Psychoses and their Response to Electroshock

It is easier to understand the progress made in the treatment of psychiatric illnesses during the past 40 years if we divide these into three main groups. The first consists of patients who have an organic disease of the brain such as that caused by a tumour or by delirium tremens. The second group comprises the psychoneuroses, or more exactly those of a milder character. The third group is that of the functional psychoses including schizophrenia and cyclothymia. The reason for this division is that the treatment of these three groups of disorders is quite different. The classical concepts of medicine and surgery are applicable to the organic group, diseases which can be treated by conventional methods. For instance, a cerebral tumour can often be removed, and delirium tremens may respond to treatment with vitamins and sedatives. Furthermore it is generally accepted that the milder neuroses should be treated by psychotherapy. Thirdly, the functional psychoses respond best to stress treatments in the form of convulsive therapy or coma treatment, or else to the application of psychotropic drugs. These drugs, like the stress treatments, have a selective action on subcortical centres which initiate and maintain both normal and pathological patterns of behaviour.

Near the beginning of this century most physicians failed to realise the radically different character of these three groups and it was widely held that the classical concept of medicine would enable psychiatrists to solve the problems of neurotic and psychotic illness. In 1870 Henry Maudsley had said (quoted by Hordern, 1958) "The observation and classification of mental disorders have been so exclusively psychological that we have not sincerely realised the fact that they illustrate the same pathological principles as other diseases, are produced in the same way, and must be investigated in the same spirit of positive research. Until this is done I see no hope of improvement in our knowledge of them and no use in multiplying books about them." Many investigators hoped to find delicate changes in the brains of schizophrenics or some germ, possibly a diphtheroid bacillus, which might be responsible. The French psychiatrist Claude suggested that schizophrenia was a neurotropic form of tuberculosis. Later it was thought that neurotic illness was the result of focal infection or even that the "nervous battery was run down". Enuresis was allegedly caused by a weak bladder. Maudsley was rightly protesting against alienists who thought only in terms of the "mind" or "soul" and of "moral insanity". He was right in the sense that we cannot understand mental disorder without a knowledge of genetics, anatomy, physiology and medicine. It was, however, still a long step from Maudsley to Adolf Meyer whose psychobiological approach was more comprehensive.

Although Maudsley's approach was suitable for the study of organic mental disease, it was not so satisfactory in regard to the psychoneuroses. It was therefore from psychiatrists of a different school that the revolutionary discovery came that the neuroses could be treated most successfully by what was called medical psychology in the 1920's. The success of analytic measures in the treatment of the neuroses encouraged Jung and Bleuler to investigate the psychology of patients suffering from early schizophrenia. Although these studies threw some light on the pathology of some schizophrenics, their therapeutic effect was negligible.

It was only in the 1930's that insulin coma and the convulsive therapies led to a second major breakthrough in psychiatric treatment, this time in the treatment of the functional psychoses. In the 1950's the discovery of chlorpromazine opened still another chapter by the introduction of the neuroleptic drugs.

Some psychiatrists still refuse to accept the view that psychotherapy is the main weapon against the neuroses but that the stress treatments and neuroleptic drugs should be used in cases of psychosis as the first part of the total treatment. Many are still using psychotherapy as their principal treatment of a typical psychosis in its initial stages, while others employ neuroleptic drugs or ECT in comparatively mild cases of neurosis. These errors can lead to serious consequences. One contributory factor to the high suicide rate is the failure of doctors to diagnose psychotic depression and to have the patient removed to hospital, where adequate

References p. 100

supervision and immediate drug or stress treatment may be given. Again it sometimes happens that an employee who is suffering from melancholia is allowed three months of sick leave in which to get better. If he is given shock treatment at the beginning he has a happy convalescence and returns to work within the allotted time. Too often however there is some procrastination, and ECT is suggested only when the period of sick leave is nearing its end, and the patient is still no better.

Some etiological considerations

Any psychiatric disorder may be considered as being the end-result of the interplay of three etiological factors, the first being that of heredity. The second factor is that of acquired injury or disease, while the third factor is that of psychological conflict, or viewed objectively, faulty conditioning and failure to adapt to the environment. Every one of these factors plays a part in each instance but the importance of each factor varies considerably from case to case. In the organic psychoses heredity may be all important as in Huntington's chorea or negligible as in cases of a cerebral tumour. In the psychoneuroses the hereditary factor is less important than in the functional psychoses. The form of psychosis with which the individual reacts to stress depends largely on his physical *habitus* and his heredity. This is shown by the work of Slater, a pupil of Rüdin (1927) who investigated hereditary prognosis. It was found that the likelihood of any one developing a particular psychosis increased according to the proximity of blood relatives who had the same disease. On the other hand the study of identical twins showed that heredity did not account entirely for the disease but that physical illness or psychological stress of a certain degree might be necessary in addition to make the disease manifest. Where one uniovular twin was affected by schizophrenia the other might escape in 22 per cent of cases (Slater, 1950).

It is possible that the inborn psychotic reaction patterns had a biological significance in the early history of mankind. For the arboreal man for instance a catatonic reaction could have been lifesaving. He would remain motionless for an indefinite period. He had a strong grasp reflex. He was without hunger and insensitive to pain, heat or cold and he retained his urine and faeces, excretion of which might have betrayed him. Such a reaction to stress, however, in the present age has no survival value, but merely constitutes a disease.

Reaction patterns in animals which are analogous to psychoses in man can be evoked in animals by quite different types of stimulus. In the monkey a catatonic-like state can be produced by administering a drug called bulbocapnine in a suitable dose. It can also be caused by excising parts of the cortex. Gantt was able to make his dog Nick catatonic by conditioning him in a special manner.

In the case of melancholia the typical syndrome can be precipitated by quite different types of stimuli. A drug such as reserpine can cause it, and Stengel (1959) has reported that it could result from specific lesions in encephalitis lethargica. Delay (1946) has described how pressure of air in the third ventricle can cause temporary symptoms of melancholia. Again, an endocrine crisis such as the menarche, pre-menstrual tension, or the menopause can be an important contributory factor.

The functional psychoses appear therefore to consist of a specific re-action pattern which is controlled at the level of the diencephalon and which can be precipitated by a non-specific stimulus.

Some characteristics of the functional psychoses

A functional psychosis is different from a typical neurosis in certain respects. The latter differs only in a quantitative rather than in a quali-tative manner from the normal. The degree of the patient's anxiety is greater, it is precipitated by a lesser stimulus and it lasts a longer time than in healthy individuals. His feelings and behaviour are more under the control of the will than are those of a psychotic patient. In the psy-chosis the hereditary factor is stronger. The patient is under the influence of an inborn reaction-pattern so that he is more controlled by his emo-tions. This is demonstrated by what patients say after treatment with electroshock. In answer to a questionnaire sent to patients a year after treatment, many replied to the question "Have there been any beneficial results from the treatment?" with the answer "The treatment gave me back my will power". From the physiological standpoint this may indicate that the individual can now act in a reasonable and logical manner at the cortical level instead of in a relatively helpless way, when his actions are perhaps more controlled at the level of the diencephalon.

It is for such reasons that we advocate applying stress treatment to the psychotic patient and in using psychotherapy and rehabilitation only after the psychotic symptoms have remitted.

Can stress treatment be useful in organic psychoses and in severe neuroses?

A surprising feature of shock treatment is that it has been found useful in treating psychotic symptoms which have been caused in part at least by organic factors. The clinical picture might be melancholic, paranoid, manic or one of confusion. The organic factor might be a toxin as in general paresis or pernicious anaemia or pellagra. Such cases have been studied by Roth and Rosie (1953) and by Fernandes and Polonio (1946) among others. It was a surprising finding that ECT could cause a re-mission of functional symptoms, even of confusion with a clouded state, and of stupor. The psychotic symptoms may be greater or less than would be expected from the organic disease and may last a longer or shorter time without reference to the latter. Treatment by electroshock may be a life-saving measure in such cases, but after the psychotic symptoms have been removed, it is still necessary to treat the organic condition which origi-nally precipitated the psychosis.

Electroshock is valuable not only in the treatment of the typical func-tional psychosis and of psychotic symptoms which occur in organic mental disorders but also in some of the psychoneuroses such as anorexia nervosa, severe hysteria and obsessional illness when these are so severe as to be obviously resistant to psychotherapy. Such conditions respond to electroshock provided it is given sufficiently early. This treatment may then make psychotherapy possible. From the point of view of treat-ment, therefore, these conditions resemble the psychoses more than they do the other neuroses.

Theoretically it is possible to treat a case of anorexia nervosa success-fully by psychotherapy at the very beginning. It appears however that there follows a further period during which the symptoms are reversible only if a stress treatment, usually ECT, is given before the psychotherapy. It is probable that a treatment suggested by Dally and Sargant (1960) of administering sub-coma insulin and a phenothiazine may be effective at a still later stage. Finally leucotomy may be necessary as a life-saving measure.

Does ECT cure the real disease?

When a patient comes to a psychiatrist with melancholia he is a very sick man. He cannot sleep, he cannot eat; he can think only about unpleasant subjects; he wants to kill himself; he cannot make decisions; he has a bad colour; he may retain his urine and faeces, and he adopts a posture of universal flexion. Yet in a typical instance, after he has received some half dozen ECT's he becomes completely symptom-free, and he may remain so for an indefinite period. Though this would seem on the face of it to be a dramatic recovery, some psychiatrists say that the symptoms may have been removed but the "real disease" has not been touched. It is worth while to examine this proposition more precisely.

As we have seen, the melancholia was the end-result of the interplay of three factors, the hereditary factor, the psychological factor and the factor of acquired physical illness. In the case of general paresis (GPI) where malaria has removed the psychological symptoms one can say that the spirochaete has not been destroyed and therefore the disease has not been cured, but in the case of the functional psychosis there is no evidence that any micro-organism has been involved. The three factors mentioned above are alone sufficient to account for the onset of the disorder.

It has been said that where a case of psychotic depression has remitted the real disease has not been touched, because there is a tendency for the symptoms to recur at a later date. The view put forward in this book however is that the clinical syndrome is in fact the disease. We are justified in claiming that the patient has recovered at least for the time being from schizophrenia when we have removed his symptoms and he feels well and has returned to work. If the clinical syndrome is not the disease, it may well be asked what is the disease? The psychoanalyst would state perhaps that the real disease is the patient's mental conflict. He might say "A sexual element entered into the son-mother relationship and this has made the patient inhibited towards the opposite sex. He has the body of a healthy man but cannot find expression for sexual activity through conventional channels and he is frustrated and retreats into the reaction-pattern of schizophrenia." It is said that he is solving his problem in his own way and that the ECT has merely removed the symptoms and left him with his original problem. There appears indeed to be an element of truth in this view. We have described elsewhere (Paterson, 1958) the case of a young woman with schizophrenic symptoms which were removed by ECT. For the time being she was "cured" but the symptoms kept recurring until she was completely changed by psychotherapy from being negatively conditioned to the opposite sex and dressing like a boy into having the feelings of a normal woman. It would be more correct however to say that at first when she had only her conflict she was a potential schizophrenic but that when she had her symptoms as well she was an overt schizophrenic. This is much clearer than to say that the real disease is the mental conflict. It should be noticed in addition that the psychotherapy would have been impossible without the previous ECT.

Again it might be said that the "real disease" is a faulty gene which occurs in the patient's family and a geneticist might predict that a certain number of cases of schizophrenia would occur in the next generation of a given family. Nevertheless for the disease to become manifest the conditions of either physical illness or mental stress or both may need to be present, as is shown by the study of uniovular twins.

If the doctrine that the symptom-complex is not the disease is true, then we may all be suffering from a multiplicity of serious diseases of which we are unaware. The fact however is that such diseases are only potential and therefore to all intents and purposes non-existent. If we equate the symptom-complex with the disease itself we remind ourselves that the condition is probably functional and therefore reversible by the newer treatments.

Diencephalic reaction patterns (DRP's)

(a) Inhibited and excited clinical pictures

If we consider functional disorders from the biological standpoint we can tabulate certain facts which are known about them as shown in the accompanying Table I. The upper part shows conditions which are predominantly inhibitory in character, while those in the bottom half are more of an excitatory charecter. It may be remarked that ECT given once or twice a week is often sufficient to bring about a remission in an inhibited state like retarded melancholia or anorexia nervosa, but in conditions like agitated melancholia, mania, or severe anxiety state with panics, ECT needs to be given in a more concentrated manner and with a greater number of applications. The same effect may be obtained by giving electronarcosis. It is convenient to refer to the functional psychoses, the functional picture in the organic psychoses, and the severer psychoneuroses, all of which are likely to respond to ECT, as diencephalic reaction patterns (DRP's).

It is of interest to note that a DRP consisting of excited behaviour can be terminated either by repeated applications of convulsions, which themselves represent a maximal state of excitation or they can be treated by maximal sedation in the form of prolonged sleep. Treatment with ECT in our experience terminates a state of mania more quickly and effectively and with fewer side effects than does chemical sedation, though admittedly phenothiazine derivatives are more commonly used.

As well as employing an electrically induced convulsion, which represents the maximal degree of stimulation, it is also possible to stimulate a limited area of the brain by externally placed electrodes in such a way as to produce a state of generalised inhibition. This is described in Chapter 6. The facilities at our disposal however have not enabled us to treat more than a limited number of patients in this way.

The inhibitory character of melancholia, apparently of the retarded type has been studied by Alexander by the conditioned reflex method (1961 a and b). The patients are subjected to the sounding of a high tone which is always associated with a painful shock to the finger, and also to a low tone which is never thus associated. In a typical case the patient after being conditioned shows only a poor response to the high tone as measured by the fall of skin resistance (if the fall is less than 2,000 ohms as here, the patient is classified as an "inhibitory type"). The patients received ECT and all 9 of them made at least a social recovery. In a period up to 6 days after the last shock treatment, the conditioned reflex was abolished. Ultimately however at the time when optimal benefits of treatment were established, there was a significant increase in the responses to the high tone from an average of 439 to an average of 1,648 ohms. The increased response in positive conditioned reflexes and also a tendency to differentiate between positive and negative signals after ECT was in line with the findings of Gellhorn (1946) who showed that ECT caused the reappearance of conditioned responses that had previously been extinguished by non-reinforcement.

References p. 100

TABLE I

SOME CHARACTERISTICS OF DIENCEPHALIC REACTION PATTERNS IN RELATION TO TREATMENT

	Time, in months, during which reversible by ECT's	Average No. of ECT's	Changes in EEG or CR?	Too few ECT's augment symptoms?	Adjunct drugs
Inhibited States					
Retarded melancholia	24+	8	CR	No	Imipramine, MAOI's
Catatonia (stuporose)	12	18	CR	No	Amylobarbitone, Phenothiazines, CO_2
Post partum depression	12+	12	CR	No	Imipramine
Anorexia nervosa	3	8–12		No	Insulin plus chlorpromazine
Obsessional inhibitions	12+	12–18		No	Perphenazine
Hysterical dissociation (paralysis etc.)	6	4–12	CR	No	Narco-analysis with amylobarbitone and methedrine
Excited States					
Mania	12	8 (concentrated at first)	EEG	Yes	Chlorpromazine
Hebephrenia	6	30–40		Yes	Phenothiazines
Agitated melancholia	6	12 (concentrated at first)		Yes	Amitryptaline plus Librium
Chronic anxiety	24+	ECT or electro-narcosis: 8–18	EEG CR	Yes	Amylobarbitone etc.
Paranoia	12+	ECT or EN: 8–18		Yes	Phenothiazines
Functional torticollis	3	EN: 12		Yes	Librium

treatments. There is no advantage in giving very concentrated treatment that will lead to incontinence. The essential point is to give a sufficient number. Hitherto some authorities have emphasised the need for sufficient insulin comas but not ECT's. A recent study (Gross et al., 1961) shows that schizophrenics who have had ECT or insulin as well as chlorpromazine remain well in a higher percentage after withdrawal of neuroleptic drugs than those who have not.

Melancholia and mania require the fewest number of treatments. Hebephrenia and catatonia the most. In excited hysterics sometimes a few ECT's have a profound effect in breaking up the dissociated state and in securing the patient's co-operation. There are, however, some hysterics with schizoid symptoms who make spectacular recoveries with some 20 treatments. One such woman who had for some years been too frightened ever to speak to anyone or go anywhere except to her office, became a professional lecturer driving her own car throughout the countryside. She had 20 ECT's. EN is equally effective.

We think that it is worth while giving ECT to cases of torticollis which are seen within the first 3 months. This is combined with psychotherapy.

We still think that ECT is the best treatment for acute mania, as the patient responds to two treatments daily within a few days and this can be spaced out later according to symptoms.

The EEG aspects of the biological "set" which forms the background of these different DRP's have been investigated by Hill (1962), Liberson (1945), Alexander (1961 a and b), Jus (1961), Meurice (1961) and others.

The last column mentions drugs commonly used to reinforce or possibly replace stress treatments. However, their effect is symptomatic rather than curative. The stress treatment stimulates the organism to terminate the morbid reaction pattern so that it is replaced by the normal pattern.

COMMENT ON TABLE I

The figures in this table are based on clinical experience and on reports in the literature and are merely intended as a basis on which more accurate work could be carried out. The table helps to present the problem of the stress treatment of different syndromes in a clearer light, showing how each disorder may be expected to respond.

The upper part of the table shows mainly inhibited syndromes. It is noticeable that they respond more rapidly and with fewer ECT's than the mainly excited syndromes in the lower half. These last are often made worse by a few ECT's but respond well if the ECT's are given more closely together (concentrated ECT) or with Electronarcosis (EN), for concentrated ECT and EN have a sedative effect on excited patients.

The first column shows roughly the time during which DRP's are reversible. There is, however, always a small percentage of longstanding cases who respond to stress treatments. I have seen a woman in California who had been a chronic mute catatonic for 30 years who passed for normal after 100 EN's.

It seems that functional torticollis can be reversed within 3 months of onset but may become chronic after that. If agitated melancholics are not treated early, they may die or be very difficult to treat.

Probably retarded melancholics and chronic anxiety states can be made to remit with ECT even after a long time. In chronic anxiety with panics EN is almost specific if combined with careful rehabilitative measures.

In the past as a rule too few treatments have been given. This has been because the technique was crude. With the co-operation of anaesthetists the treatment is maximally effective and easy on the patient. Curves like those of Danziger show how essential it is to give an adequate number of

References p. 100

(b) The reversibility of psychoses by ECT

It appears that differences exist between one psychosis and another in regard to the period during which it is reversible by the application of electroshock treatment. Many writers have produced statistics which show that proportionally more schizophrenic patients recover, the earlier in the disease treatment is given (see Figs. 2, 3 and 4). The first column in Table I gives the approximate period during which ECT is likely to be effective. It is based partly on our own figures and partly on those of others.

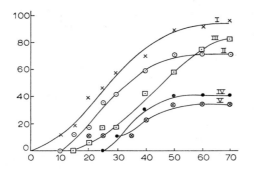

Fig. 2. Outcome of adequate electric shock therapy in dementia praecox. Ordinate, percentage of courses of treatment ending in recovery of patient. Abscissa, cumulative number of treatments. Mean duration of illness before treatment, by groups: I, 3.0 months; II, 7.6 months; III, 15.0 months; IV, 36.0 months; V, 105.5 months.

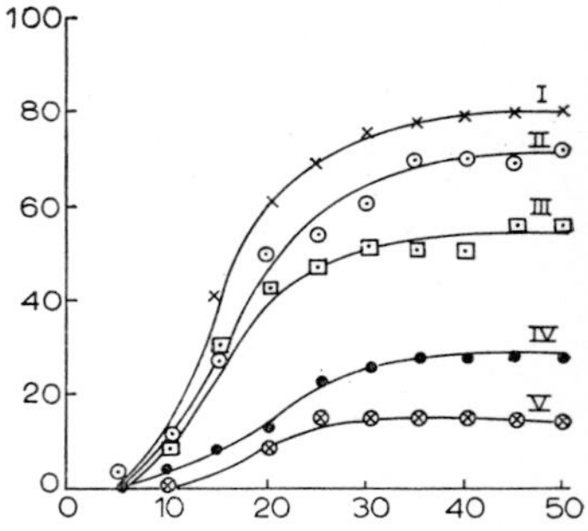

Fig. 3. Outcome of adequate insulin shock therapy in dementia praecox. Ordinate, percentage of courses of treatment ending in recovery of patient. Abscissa, cumulative number of insulin comas. Mean duration of illness before first treatment, by groups: I, 3.0 months; II, 8.0 months; III, 16.7 months; IV, 37.0 months; V, 96 months (Danziger and Kindwall, 1946).

The situation with regard to recurrent melancholia however is more debatable. At the Cambridge Symposium on Depression 1959, it was suggested that in some cases of depression, there was a period at the beginning of the illness where the patient was refractory to ECT and that the refractory state gradually diminished over a period of some weeks or months. It was said that the psychiatrist should hold his hand and give ECT only when the period of recovery was beginning. In our experience however almost every case will react to ECT at the beginning. If the patient is very agitated he may need 2 a day for 2 days but this is rare. In most of the bad cases 1 a day for 3 days is sufficient, followed by a treatment every other day for some 6 more treatments. The patient can then have 2 a week or 1 a week depending on his response. Nowadays the addition of imipramine will shorten the duration of treatment. We have had a number of cases of recurrent depression where attacks which usually lasted 3 months have now been reduced to 10 days. Russell *et al.* (1953) urged the use of more intense ECT generally.

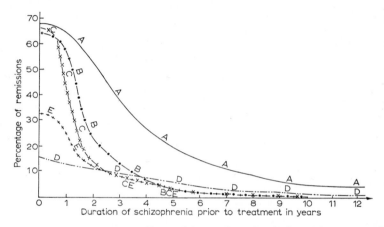

Fig. 4. Comparing the therapeutic effects of largactil, with which ECT was generally combined, A; Deep insulin, B; Convulsive therapy, C; Leucotomy operation, D; and routine hospitalisation, E; (Blair and Brady, 1958).

It may be noted from the diagram (Fig. 2) that nearly twice as many patients recover from schizophrenia if 30 or 40 electric treatments are given to a patient who has been ill for 3 months than if only 15 are given. The same holds for those who have been ill for 7 months. The same trends are present for insulin coma treatment (Fig. 3). About twice as many of those who have been ill less than 3 months recover after 60 comas as after 25.

In the past at some hospitals the technique of giving ECT has not been ideal and long courses have been difficult because of the onset of transitory confusion and euphoria. It is likely that it is the number of treatments which is important and not the concentration of treatments. Nevertheless, concentration is often necessary in a case of agitated melancholia in order

References p. 100

to terminate as rapidly as possible symptoms which are dangerous to life.

(c) Number of treatments necessary to effect a remission in a diencephalic reaction pattern (DRP)

Table I shows that certain psychoses are more resistant to the effects of ECT than others. Melancholia, especially the retarded variety, responds with a smaller number of treatments than does schizophrenia. It was this characteristic of depression which led some psychiatrists to exaggerate the alleged specificity of ECT in the treatment of melancholia. Arnold and Hoff (1961) have shown for instance that certain forms of schizophrenia are just as susceptible to the effects of ECT as melancholia. Fig. 2 shows how the more resistive forms of psychosis do yield in time to ECT if a sufficient number of treatments are given (Danziger and Kindwall, 1946). There is a fair degree of agreement that if insulin coma is given in schizophrenia, the number of complete cures as opposed to social recoveries is a little higher than in the case of ECT where only a short course is given. There is also evidence that insulin-treated patients stay well for a longer time. It is likely however that this difference depends more on the quantity of treatment given rather than on a qualitative difference. It has been the custom in many hospitals to give as many as 40 or even 100 insulin comas but a maximum of only 10 or 20 ECT's. In some cases the reason for this has been faulty technique in giving the ECT. Treatment has been stopped because of confusional and manic symptoms which could have been avoided.

Another quantitative difference between electroshock and insulin coma is that on each occasion the insulin coma lasts for a longer time than the coma caused by shock. Where the coma caused by ECT has been prolonged by subconvulsive stimulation (electronarcosis technique) the therapeutic effects have been better. Monro (1950) has given statistics of remissions in schizophrenia from electronarcosis treatment which were superior to those obtained in the state of New York in schizophrenia treated by insulin coma (see Chapter 4, p. 52).

(d) The principle of mutual incompatibility between different DRP's

The reason why Meduna introduced convulsive therapy in the treatment of schizophrenia was that he believed epilepsy to be antagonistic to schizophrenia. Meduna (1937) spoke of a biological antagonism between the two disorders. However Hoch (1943) maintained that the two disorders are neither opposed to each other nor related to each other. He bases his findings on clinical, genetic and electroencephalographic considerations. The concept of incompatibility however between one psychotic or psychoneurotic reaction pattern and another remains a valuable one.

Conditions in animals such as bulbocapnine intoxication in monkeys which imitate psychotic states in man, show in a striking manner how one "psychosis" is incompatible with another. If one gradually increases the dose of bulbocapnine one obtains successively 4 different "psychotic" pictures. At first the animal is inactive or moves slowly with hanging head as if depressed. With a larger dose however he passes into a condition resembling catatonia. A grasp reflex appears and the monkey will hang by one forepaw from a bar for a lengthy period. This does not occur in the normal animal. When the dosage is further increased the monkey goes into a state of mania and with a higher dosage still he has epileptic convulsions (Richter and Paterson, 1931 and 1932). This experiment shows that there are clear-cut reaction patterns which are controlled at the level of the diencephalon and which are mutually exclusive, the picture suddenly changing completely with a small increase in the dosage of the drug.

From the clinical standpoint it appears that some psychoses are incompatible with others. Melancholic symptoms are not found in hebephrenic patients. A state of mania is also incompatible with schizophrenic symptoms. One patient, a man of 40, developed schizophrenia and did not speak to anybody for 10 years because he believed that he could read every one else's thoughts and that every one could read what he was thinking. For that reason speech seemed unnecessary. However in time he was coaxed to work in the hospital garden. For some reason, possibly related to his new activity, he developed a manic reaction. This took the place of his schizophrenic reaction and when the mania remitted he remained normal and was able to return home.

It has often been remarked by psychiatrists that the prognosis in schizophrenia is better if the clinical picture keeps changing, especially if there is an admixture of depressive or manic symptoms. When that happens there is more chance of the clinical picture returning permanently to a state of normality.

References p. 100

(e) Neurophysiological aspects of the DRP

We have referred to the functional psychosis as a reaction pattern of the nervous system. Meurice (1961) and others talk of a "bioelectric homeostasis" which is different in each psychosis. Meurice has compared the reactions of schizophrenics to those of normals under experimental conditions. The subject for investigation lies in a quiet dark room and his reactions to various stimuli are tested. A record is made of the EEG (particularly the alpha rhythm), the EKG, the skin resistance and muscle tone. The various stimuli to which the individual is subjected indicate either danger or a state of tranquility to him. The stimuli again may induce fatigue or sleep by constant repetition. It was found that schizophrenics react quite differently from normals when examined in this way. In normals there is much more alpha rhythm during the resting state. In schizophrenics the heart rate is frequently outside normal limits, being either abnormally rapid or abnormally slow. Normal subjects show more hypertonus of muscle in response to an alerting signal and they show more signs of fatigue as well as more reactivity in the EEG and skin resistance.

Alexander (1961 a and b) who has described how faulty conditioning in melancholia becomes normal after ECT, has also studied conditioning in cases of anxiety neurosis and in schizophrenia. In the former condition the subject reacts to a neutral stimulus with almost the same degree of fear reaction as to the auditory stimulus which is associated with danger. After successful treatment however this failure to differentiate disappears.

Despite the abnormalities described by Meurice (1961) in the reactivity of schizophrenics, Alexander found that they could be conditioned to react to a danger signal as readily as normals. In this respect they differ from cases of anxiety neurosis and of melancholia.

Studies such as those of Meurice and of Alexander give us a clearer picture of the internal milieu or "l'homéostase bioélectrique" which characterises the psychosis and which can suddenly be terminated by shock treatment and replaced by the bioelectric homeostasis of the normal individual. It is likely that in the future this type of investigation will throw more light on the nature of the functional psychoses.

(f) The psychobiological approach to the functional psychoses

It has been said that there is as yet no common basis on which the majority of psychiatrists would agree — a basis on which one could build a theory regarding the pathology and treatment of mental disorders. The holistic philosophy of Adolf Meyer however is perhaps the most satisfying for this purpose. In his account of psychobiology, Meyer contended that living man should be studied as a whole person in action, that is, as an integrated organism whose functions are arranged in a hierarchical manner. Although man is the indivisible unit of study, he can be considered from any one of a number of hierarchically arranged levels. Beginning at the base one can study the physics and chemistry of the cell unit. At a higher level the physiologist studies the functioning of parts of the body but the investigation of the whole person in action is the work of the psychobiologist. The patient is studied as it were in cross section on a particular day. In addition a full "longitudinal" record is made of the patient's physical and psychological development from his birth to the present time. This includes his psychosexual development and his social adaptation.

Meyer's approach to the patient was essentially a humanistic one. Successful treatment in the last resort depended on persuading the patient to make the best possible adaptation to his environment. Where rapport was possible between doctor and patient Meyer would say (see Muncie, 1959) "The patient comes with his own view of his trouble; the physician has another view. Treatment consists of the joint effort to bring about that approximation of views which will be the most effective in the situation."

This attitude however applies only when the psychiatrist is dealing with a patient with whom he is in rapport. When the patient is psychotic however, one could not in a typical case reason with him in this manner. Under such circumstances the psychobiologist is compelled to apply treatment at a lower level than that at which one can reason with a patient. Only when the symptoms are removed in this fashion can psychotherapy be applied. Some Meyerians were slow to appreciate the value of shock treatment but Meyer himself could see no theoretical objection to the use of leucotomy and still less, no doubt, to the employment of shock therapy.

Meyer was not content to approach his patients entirely from the subjective point of view and to rely solely on what the patient told him. He said that people were judged by their behaviour and that behaviour could be studied objectively. Behaviour at the highest human level could be influenced by instinctive reactions at a lower level which were not always conscious. It was possibly such considerations that led Meyer to put J. B. Watson the Behaviourist in charge of his laboratory at the John Hopkins Hospital. The two biologists who have been influenced by Watson and who have worked at the Phipps Clinic since Watson's time have both contributed greatly to the understanding of the pathology of the functional psychoses. Richter (1931) has shown how the endocrine glands can influence spontaneous activity and how fluctuations of the latter are closely related to cyclothymia. He has studied conditions resembling psychosis in man which are produced in monkeys by bulbocapnine. He has shown how recurrent psychotic states are analogous to physiological cycles which occur in animals. Both are reaction patterns involving the autonomic nervous system and the endocrine system and are controlled at the diencephalic level. Again, Gantt has shown the significance of the conditioned reflex approach to psychiatry. He has described how conditioning of a certain kind can lead in time to a psychotic state in the dog (1950). The multi-dimensional or psychobiological approach to treatment has been discussed by the author elsewhere (Paterson, 1958).

Mode of action of electrocerebral treatment

In 1948 in a lecture to the Psychiatric Section of the Royal Society of Medicine I gave an account of the *modus operandi* of electrocerebral treatment (Paterson, 1948 c). Since then I have seen no reason to alter what I said at that time. The following is an account of what I said. "Adolf Meyer's doctrine of reaction types has proved on the whole to be a valuable one. He speaks, for instance, of the catatonic, the manic, the melancholic, or the chronically anxious patient, as having reacted to environmental stress by adopting a special type of reaction. Meyer thought of this reaction type as being modifiable by treatment such as rest, or by withdrawing the patient to the quiet of hospital under a sympathetic and understanding physician who could influence him at the conscious level.

The remarkable and unexpected success however of these recent physiological treatments in the psychoses or intractable psychoneuroses suggests that we must visualise the morbid reaction type as depending on a particular reaction pattern or "set" of the autonomic nervous system and the endocrine system, controlled at the level of the diencephalon.

It has been found that such reaction patterns may be produced experimentally by certain drugs. Bulbocapnine, for instance, in ascending doses will produce in the macac monkey first depression of activity, then catalepsy, then a state resembling mania, and finally epilepsy. Again, Gjessing (1938) has shown that recurrent catatonia can result from faulty protein metabolism.

Although such reaction patterns can sometimes be produced by drugs, it is of course usual for environmental stress to be a factor in their causation. The particular morbid reaction pattern depends no doubt to a considerable degree on heredity, but imitation and suggestion can in some cases be the determining cause as shown by epidemics of hysteria in the Middle Ages or by the fact that the American negro shows different clinical pictures from his African cousin (Carothers, 1947).

If therefore the physiological basis of a commencing psychosis consists of a particular "set" or pattern of the nervous system, it is necessary to attempt immediately to alter this "set" by these electrical means. If the stupor, melancholia, mania or severe anxiety is allowed to continue, the condition may become intractable, or some complication such as suicide, inanition or intercurrent disease may ensue.

The electric current does not, we suppose, effect a recovery merely by its convulsant action, but by the autonomic changes which occur during the coma which accompanies and outlasts the convulsion. This perhaps explains why electronarcosis is more effective than electroshock.

The passage of an electric current is not merely a way of frightening the patient at the conscious level, like throwing a broody hen into a pond. It is true that the ancients thought that thy cured some madmen by throwing them into the sea from a cliff. Medieval monks held the heads of the insane under water till the priest had completed his prayer. Erasmus Darwin spun them round in a revolving chair and at Bethlem the patients were made to fall through a trapdoor into a cold bath. In the present treatment however the patient is usually first anaesthetised and the treatment is carried out, as stated, entirely at the unconscious level. There is therefore no question of the treatment taking effect by the patient being subjected to conscious fear.

If this view is correct, then it is imperative to treat these patients as soon as the morbid state is manifest, a fact which is borne out by the higher proportion of successes with early psychotic cases. The time for rest and psychotherapy in these severe cases is after the electrocerebral treatment and not before.

Some psychiatrists still hesitate to carry out these treatments at an early stage in patients who are obviously too ill for psychotherapy, because of possible injury to their brains. It is a fact nevertheless that in the hundreds of cases treated no complaint has been made by any patient or his relatives of any serious side-effect of the treatment.

We are still unable to explain why patients look and feel so much better after a few treatments, or why chronic skin diseases should clear up. Cerletti, for instance, told me that he brought about a recovery in 14 out of 16 cases of psoriasis by means of electroshock. His theory that the brain develops a specific substance when threatened with approaching death is still unproved. It may be however that these remarkable changes are effected in part by endocrine means, particularly through the pituitary."

Since 1948 some of these statements have been borne out by the work of others. Roth and Rosie (1953) have pointed out that the suddenness with which the morbid symptoms are replaced in some cases by the normal state suggests that ECT is acting on a controlling centre. Roth (1951) has also described EEG changes relating to the hypothalamus which occur in response to pentothal, generally after the fourth ECT, which are coincidental with improvement in the patient's condition. This improvement includes physical as well as mental changes. His appetite and sleep improve and he loses his sallow complexion.

The work of Selye (1957) has thrown some light on how a non-specific stressor can bring about a remission in a disease by producing a stress reaction in the organism. He calls this reaction "The General Adaptation Syndrome" (GAS).

He has demonstrated that a stressor causes marked changes in the hypothalamus which in time affects the pituitary gland, more especially the anterior lobe. The GAS consists of three stages: the alarm reaction, the stage of resistance and the stage of exhaustion. Although all the organs of the body are involved in the process, a change of the integration of the endocrine nervous system is the central phenomenon.

The threat which the ECT signifies for the organism brings into play the alarm reaction which consists of two successive phases; the first resembles that of surgical shock in which there is a fall of blood pressure and of temperature. There is a concentration of the blood and a rise of calcium content. A transitory rise of blood sugar is followed by a subsequent fall. There is a leucopenia which is followed by leucocytosis and eosinopenia. In this phase the anti-inflammatory hormones, ACTH and cortisone, are predominant. In the counter-shock phase which follows however, there is a rise of blood sugar and the pro-inflammatory hormones, STH (somatotrophic hormone), aldosterone and DOC (desoxy-corticosterone) are active. The harmonious progress of general adaptation however does not always occur in response to stress, for other hormones or nervous reactions from specific conditioning can cause a derailment of the process. In most cases however the GAS is brought to a successful conclusion. In addition to the hypothalamic-pituitary mechanism referred to above, other hormones may also be secreted, such as acetylcholine, histamine, anti-histamines and sympathin.

It seems from Selye's description that the ultimate effect of the stressor is to terminate the state of equilibrium or homeostasis which characterises the functional psychosis, and to replace it by another form of homeostasis, which is that of normality. It is of interest that the application of stress can have the additional effect of causing the disappearance of concomitant diseases such as skin infections. It is also of interest that the psychotic reaction pattern which accompanies an organic disease such as pernicious anaemia or syphilis can be terminated by ECT even although the organic disease persists, as pointed out by Roth and Rosie (1953). For a fuller account of the effects of ECT on the endocrine systems and cerebral nervous systems see Ashby (1952) and Pronko et al. (1960).

Mode of action of the phenothiazines

At the Colloquium at Paris in 1955 Delay (1956) contrasted the effects of chlorpromazine with those of ECT. The latter causes an alarm reaction in which the defensive mechanisms of the body are mobilised, whereas the phenothiazines have from the beginning a calming effect.

The action of drugs on the nervous system will be dealt with in a later

Chapter but is is worth noting at this point that they resemble ECT in the following respects. They act on the diencephalon (the meso-diencephalic activating system) and centres closely connected with it. In this way they also influence the feeling tone related to a particular psychic disorder. They differ from shock treatments however in that they must be continued for an indefinite time in most cases. The diencephalon occupies a key position in the whole autonomic and endocrine systems. It regulates the adaptation of the organism to the environment through the continuation of an internal equilibrium or homeostasis. This homeostasis can be influenced by drugs which act chiefly at one of four different points: (i) the cortex; (ii) the limbic system; (iii) the hypothalamus; and (iv) the mid-brain reticular substance.

Thus far we have been concerned mainly with the historical and theoretical background of our subject. In subsequent Chapters we shall describe the actual techniques which are subsumed under the term electro-cerebral treatments, namely, electroconvulsive therapy (ECT), electronarcosis, electrical anaesthesia, electrically induced sleep and electrically induced abreaction. We must first consider however, the requirements for a suitable machine for carrying out these treatments.

CHAPTER 2

Types of Machine and the Technique of ECT

The following qualities are looked for by most psychiatrists in an electro-shock machine at the present time. It should be simple, easy and quick to use and it should be foolproof. It should be light and easily portable. It should be of simple construction and able to stand up to a certain amount of rough usage, such as being shaken up in a motor car. One should be sure of causing a convulsion and not merely stunning the patient. On the other hand there should be a minimal loss of memory or confusion in the patient.

Most machines use AC current from the mains. There is some evidence that a diphasic current is less injurious to the brain than a unidirectional one, unless in the latter case one frequently changes the polarity. Lilly *et al.* (1955) found more damage to a monkey's brain after repeated electroshocks given over a period of weeks with a unidirectional pulse current than with a diphasic current. They also found that with AC the threshold for the convulsion became lower with each application, but the contrary was the case with the unidirectional current. Physiologists are agreed that it is the strength of the current which is important and not the voltage or electrical energy applied to the brain.

It is known that the ability of a machine to cause a convulsion depends on the duration of the current as well as its strength. If therefore a certain voltage is just subliminal for one second it will effect a convulsion if the current is held for a second or two more (Paterson, 1946).

Some psychiatrists speak as if no harm can be done if a high current is passed through the brain but this is not our experience. We have encountered patients who have complained of symptoms resembling those of surgical shock and accompanied by severe headache, and on occasion we have found that an exceptionally high current has been used. This occurred when the resistance at the electrodes was made as low as possible during an experiment. Again one of our patients who came from a foreign

References p. 100

country had these symptoms every time she received a shock treatment there but when she received a liminal shock in our clinic she had no such symptoms.

We prefer to use a machine which has an ammeter so that one can read the current directly (Paterson, 1960). This is a more scientific procedure because it is on the strength of the current that the physiological changes depend. Many Italian psychiatrists use this type of machine. One can control the strength of current merely by the manual rotation of a switch. It is only with this type of machine that one can apply the techniques of electronarcosis or subconvulsive electrical abreaction described in this book in addition to electroshock.

We also employ on occasion an apparatus which can deliver a uni-directional pulse current with a square shaped or saw-tooth current. With this last machine one can vary the frequency, the duration of the pulse and the intensity of the current. This is the machine which is used in physiological work where it is desirable that the stimulation be uniform. If it is important to obtain a good therapeutic effect in treating a psychotic patient but at the same time to reduce to a minimum the memory loss, then in our experience the best technique is to use a unidirectional pulse current placing the cathode on the vertex and the anode low down on the motor area, after the administration of an anaesthetic. The procedure is then repeated on the opposite side. In this way the patient obtains a good "lift" but does not suffer memory loss even with a large number of applications. The reason is that with liminal currents the stimulation is confined almost entirely to the cathode area, the part round the anode being relatively unaffected. Nevertheless there is the usual physiological spread of the impulse to the subcortical trigger area to produce a fit.

For those who require an apparatus where no mains supply is available, machines are on the market which can be worked from a battery.

Technique of premedication: Nowadays many patients receiving ECT are also being treated with chlorpromazine. It is dangerous however to treat a patient who is having high doses of the drug. It is nevertheless safe to give ECT to a patient who has had not more thans 150 mg of chlorpromazine, or 100 mg of tofranil, during the previous day. In such cases the blood pressure should be examined before treatment. Since the advent of scoline it is necessary to be much more strict in seeing that the patient's stomach is completely empty, for this drug relaxes the cardiac sphincter, thus allowing fluids to flow back into the mouth.

Premedication consists first of all in the injection of atropine, 1/75 of a grain i.m. (1 mg i.m.), three quarters of an hour before the treatment. This reduces drastically the secretion of mucus or saliva, and prevents over-action of the vagus in slowing the heart or lowering the blood pressure. Needless to say it does not abolish the secretions which are already there. The air passages must always be cleared and septic foci dealt with prior to the treatment. It is strange that some writers think that atropine is unnecessary and it is said that the patients object to having a dry mouth. However Clement (1962) has shown that if atropine 1 mg is given i.v. 75 sec before treatment there is no disturbance of circulation but if it is given subcutaneously 30 min before there can be a marked fall of blood pressure (systolic reaching below 100 mm of Hg) for 5 sec after the ECT. As will be shown later in discussing the dangers of ECT, atropine is essential to give the patient maximal protection. Hargreaves (1962) shows that the intravenous route is preferable. It is efficient in preventing excessive salivation; it also obviates the patient becoming very anxious prior to treatment.

Pentothal is the drug most commonly used as an i.v. anaesthetic (see also p. 47). Nowadays it is given in 2.5 per cent concentration and therefore in a 20-ml syringe. This greatly diminishes the irritation caused to the tissues should the drug escape from the vein; its physiological effects too can be more easily controlled. The vomiting centre is not stimulated as occurs with some other anaesthetics. Intra-cranial tension is reduced. It is destroyed in the liver and hence if that organ is diseased anaesthesia will be prolonged. Furthermore it lowers the blood pressure. It is contra-indicated in very old people and in those suffering from severe circulatory disturbances or anaemia or in diseases of the liver or kidneys. The usual dose is about 200 mg. Pentothal abolishes the effect of the catecholamines as shown by Havens et al. (1959). It is of interest that adrenaline and noradrenaline were originally increased after each ECT in a large group of patients but the administration of pentothal greatly reduced the degree of elevation, thus showing that this phenomenon had no therapeutic value.

Workers in the U.S.A. are nervous about the use of pentothal and give

References p. 100

it in comparatively low doses. Many prefer to give a short-acting anaesthetic (surital, transithal). This incidentally enables the worker to treat a greater number of patients during one session. The disadvantage however arises if an anxious patient wakes up early, because he would be less likely to be calm than if his sleep lasted a longer time. Fifty mg chlorpromazine i.m. prolongs the action of pentothal by some hours.

The use of scoline (suxamethonium chloride, B.P. add.):   This was introduced into Britain towards the end of 1951 by Scurr, and its action in ECT was fully discussed by Edridge (1952). It is no exaggeration to say that the use of this drug has changed the whole character of treatment by electroshock. Before its introduction, our patients had been treated by other relaxants. In many cases the use of such drugs did not cause very much relaxation of muscles. There was often considerable trouble with cyanosis. The whole treatment caused more stress and strain on the patients and they were less willing to continue with the treatment. The use of scoline made it much easier to give a larger number of treatments without unpleasant side-effects and in this way the range of psychiatric conditions which could be successfully treated was widened. It is remarkable that the value of scoline was not appreciated by many psychiatric writers for a long time. One can still read in certain textbooks that it is sufficient to hold the patient down to prevent the occurrence of fractures or that the use of scoline adds another danger of a fatality.

Before the advent of scoline the chief danger came from the initial "jack-knife contraction" of the spine. This contraction is caused by the electric current stimulating the pyramidal tracts at the level of the internal capsule. There is also a violent contraction of the thighs. It is at this stage that a lumbar vertebra may be crushed in unpremedicated ECT or in a few cases that the head of the femur, possibly on both sides, can be driven through the acetabulum.

It was unfortunate that such complications were most likely to occur in muscular individuals, who were most incapacitated by them. The use of scoline however has prevented the development of such complications.

Attempts have been made to soften the effect of the shock on the muscles by various electrical devices. The so-called glissando modification was given. In this case the current was gradually increased within the period of a second so that the jack-knife contraction was not so pronounced. However, since a fracture can occur during either the tonic phase which follows the jack-knife contraction or the clonic phase, this procedure is inadequate. Other methods employed have been to give the patient an initial sub-convulsive shock which has the effect of lowering muscle tone for the time being, and also, instead of using a current of high intensity for a short time, to use a current of relatively low intensity for a longer time. None of these electrical procedures however had the effect of lowering very much the incidence of fractures. Some writers advocated the passage of a current through the brain during the clonic phase but the effect of this was merely to increase the tone of the muscles during the intervals between the clonic contractions. It was in fact quite a useless procedure.

The action of scoline on muscles: Normally the sequence of events initiated by a nerve impulse may be summarised as follows. The arrival of the impulse at the nerve endings causes a release of acetylcholine which depolarises the membrane of the motor end-plate. This generates an end-plate potential which in turn initiates a propagated excitation of the muscle fibre, leading to its contraction. The released acetylcholine is then rapidly hydrolysed by the enzyme cholinesterase so that the depolarisation caused by a single nerve-impulse does not persist beyond the refractory period of the muscle fibre, and a second wave of excitation does not occur (Montagu, 1953). Whereas curare has the effect of saturating the receptors at the muscle membrane and thus preventing acetylcholine from acting on them, scoline acts in quite a different manner (Hobson and Prescott, 1949). It acts rather like a large and prolonged dose of acetylcholine itself by depolarising first the muscle membrane, and this causes the familiar fibrillary twitching seen clinically. It also depolarises a narrow zone of underlying muscle tissue. The acetylcholine finds these muscles already depolarised and they remain so for some three minutes, so that the acetylcholine cannot take effect. Eventually however the scoline is hydrolysed by cholinesterase probably into succinic acid and choline which occur naturally in the body and are non-toxic.

The chief danger of giving scoline is that in certain patients there may be an undue delay in recovery from the effects of scoline. Ordinarily the effects of scoline are complete within a period of some three minutes. In one case in two thousand however there is prolonged apnoea. If however one never exceeds the equivalent of 30 mg to a 70 kg man, then such a complication will never be fatal, provided oxygenation is kept up. In these cases there is a low level of cholinesterase and pseudo-cholinesterase in the blood. The effect of this is that the scoline in the blood is not hydrolysed and therefore made ineffective. At the moment there is no known antidote to scoline but if oxygen insufflation is kept up then respiration will be restored.

The advantages of scoline are that it has a rapid action, is of brief duration and that there is a relative lack of secondary effects. We have now used it for some nine years and it would seem to be the almost ideal muscular relaxant for shock therapy. Scoline can however cause painful contraction of the muscles when its action begins, and for this reason pentothal is given first from a different syringe, but through the same needle. With the use of scoline, up to twelve patients can be treated in an hour without undue haste. Some would even put the figure at fifteen. This compares with six patients per hour treated with flaxedil and four with *d*-tubocurarine.

It sometimes happens that the point of the needle comes out of the vein and that the scoline is injected by mistake into the tissues. This may lead to an accident through the scoline not taking effect. It is therefore advisable to watch whether fibrillation has occurred before giving the shock. Again if the drug has been injected into the tissues, there may be a delayed action. This is seldom dangerous but it causes the patient some apprehension and discomfort from dyspnoea. It is unlikely that the patient will require more oxygen. All that is necessary is reassurance that the disagreeable sensations will soon pass.

The use of oxygen: During the apnoeic period oxygen is administered by intermittent manual positive pressure. Generally an inflatable rubber bag is used but others prefer the use of insufflation-bellows. An oxygen cylinder can be attached to the bellows but some anaesthetists merely use air except in an extreme emergency. Care should be taken to see that the oxygen pressure does not exceed 15 mm of mercury. Excessive pressure has been known to cause rupture of the lungs, or the air may pass more into the stomach than into the lungs. The chin should be well tilted upwards. In cases of prolonged apnoea the oxygen has to be administered over a long period of time and this proves satisfactory as long as the pulse remains of good quality. If the pulse becomes feeble the best procedure is to give rhythmical artificial respiration with oxygen. The movement of the chest aids the circulation and the pulse soon becomes strong again.

The emergency tray: Among other things it should have (1) ampoules of nikethamide 2 ml for i.v. injection, (2) airways, (3) blood pressure apparatus, (4) an intubation set, (5) more than one oxygen cylinder, (6) a suction apparatus, (7) a tongue forceps and (8) a tourniquet.

The precautions to be taken in the technique are mostly referred to in the subsequent Chapter on Complications. It may be said here however that accidents would be rarer if the following precautions were taken:

(i) A full history, particularly of physical illnesses, should be obtained.

(ii) If the patient has recently been on corticosteroid therapy he must resume it and he must be given 100 mg hydrocortisone i.v. half-an-hour before treatment.

(iii) Caution should be exercised if the thyroid gland is enlarged, and the treatment is probably contra-indicated if there is thyro-toxicosis.

(iv) There should be no sign of thrombotic veins because of the danger of infarction.

(v) The stomach should be completely empty of fluid or solid matter.

(vi) The mouth should be absolutely clean and free of mucus or infections.

(vii) There should be no loose teeth and no dentures.

(viii) Not more than 30 mg of scoline should be used and the minimal dose of pentothal for the particular patient given in 0.25 per cent solution of water.

(ix) Artificial respiration should be steady and continuous and the patient under scoline must not be left with his chest not moving.

(x) A finger should always be on the patient's pulse.

(xi) It is often beneficial to raise the foot of the bed if the patient's condition is giving rise to anxiety. On the whole one should be cautious with patients who appear to be nervous and frightened of the treatment.

(xii) The operator must be particularly dexterous in the use of syringes and needles. It is easier to find a vein if the patient has had an injection of largactil the night before and also if the limb has been warmed in hot water or by the apposition of a hot water bottle (see Veterans Administration, 1956).

References p. 100

CHAPTER 3

Complications of Electroshock Treatment and their Prevention

For the psychiatrist who is learning to give electrocerebral treatment the list of accidents in the published literature seems at first sight to be formidable. This impression however is misleading, as the majority of accidents occurred before the introduction of a short-acting muscular relaxant in the form of suxamethonium chloride B.P. (scoline, anectine). In Britain the fullest account of deaths caused by electrocerebral treatment was given in the Presidential Address to the Psychiatric Section of the Royal Society of Medicine by W. S. Maclay (1953), who was a senior commissioner of the Board of Control. Maclay's cases were included in a fuller study by Impastato in 1957. The majority of these deaths occurred as a result of cardiovascular attacks and fractures. Even if these deaths could not have been avoided before the advent of muscle relaxants, deaths from other causes could nearly all have been prevented. In almost no case was an anaesthetist present. In many instances a long-acting muscular relaxant, such as tubocurarine or flaxedil was used and it appears that frequently these patients were not given assistance with an effective respiratory apparatus. In yet other cases the patient was stated to be either aged and infirm,, and a calculated risk was taken on account of the serious nature of the mental disorder which was threatening the patient's life. Sometimes an inadequate physical examination had been carried out. In some cases laboratory tests which were in fact indicated had not been carried out. The toll of deaths related by Maclay reflected the lack of organisation and initiative necessary to give the psychiatric invalid an equal chance with the surgical patient.

Some complications caused by electroshock are briefly discussed in this chapter, but it must be realised that the advent of scoline therapy has made the occurrence of most of them practically impossible. Before the use of scoline, bone injuries included compression fractures of lumbar vertebrae, which, although usually slight, occurred with a frequency of one in ten cases. Since the introduction of treatment with scoline however, which has been used in our clinic since 1952, there has not been any serious accident. We have never, since the beginning of electroshock treatment, had any death attributable to the treatment.

In 1957 a male patient at a London mental hospital had both heads of femurs driven through the acetabula, and finding himself permanently injured, sued the hospital responsible. This accident decided Barker and Baker (1959) to investigate psychiatric practice in giving ECT. At this time medical opinion was divided as to whether muscle relaxants had any real advantages. Barker and Baker found that in the London area only 60 per cent of hospitals used thiopentone and muscle relaxants. Rather surprisingly 25 per cent used relaxants without pentothal — a practice which causes unnecessary distress to the patient, unless one uses Impastato's (1956) device of giving a sub-shock as an anaesthetic. The British Medical Association has recently recommended that scoline should not be given except by an anaesthetist, and yet it was found in the present study that an anaesthetist was employed at fewer than half the hospitals around London; in about half, treatment was given by a psychiatric Registrar working single handed. Accidents, however, have been remarkably rare. Up to the time of Barker and Baker's study, in over a quarter of a million cases there were only 9 deaths, the average age of the victims being 67, and 6 of the 9 were calculated risks, who had pre-existing disease of a grave character. One death was caused by giving excessive chlorpromazine during the course of treatment by electroplexy.

One fact which emerges from this study is the need, if the maximum safety in electroshock treatment is to be ensured, for psychiatrists to be aided by an anaesthetist wherever possible, or else to undergo a special course in anaesthetics, as do some general practitioners.

Complications

Cardio-vascular complications

A number of cases of so-called cardiac failure have been reported, especially if a current has been given which is of high intensity and long duration. If the electrodes are placed far back on the temples it is possible that an accident may be caused by a slowing or arrest of the heart from vagal stimulation. The injection of 1 mg (1/75 grain) of atropine i.m. will prevent this complication. Again, if too much pentothal is given too quickly there may be an inhibition of the heart which again can be counteracted by the administration of atropine. This accident is more likely to happen if the drug is given through a large needle and this is more frequently done in the case of young muscular men. In some parts of the world it is illegal to give pentothal without atropine.

Cardiovascular complications are reviewed by Perrin (1961). In unmodified ECT there is a sequence of vagal, sympathetic, vagal and again sympathetic predominance. The first vagal action is very brief but causes a fall of blood pressure and slowing of the heart. It is abolished by atropine and it is probably caused by stimulation of the vagus as it leaves the skull. This is immediately followed by a rise in blood pressure and a rapid heart during the tonic-clonic phase. This effect begins to diminish towards the end of the clonus and the second vagal period corresponds to the hypotonic stage with areflexia but rises again during the hypertonic phase of "decerebration". Since the systolic blood pressure can rise as high as 250 mm of Hg, a ganglion blocking agent such as beparon* could be used to prevent an excessive rise; this is not done often enough in practice (Davies and Paterson, 1952). Muscle relaxants have little effect in modifying the rise in blood pressure, but a curious phenomenon which we have noted is that a subconvulsive stimulus lowers it. In unmodified ECT the venous pressure may rise to 80 mm Hg but scoline reduces this to only a few mm Hg.

Cardiac output

The effect of modifying ECT is to diminish the cardiac output during the seizure but this is followed by an increased output. There is hardly any rise in the level of lactic acid in the blood owing to the muscle paralysis. Oxygen consumption is much less. The blood flow is greatly increased through the brain and 30 sec after the fit, the blood flow through the brain is nearly 250 per cent of normal. There is a preferential flow to the

---

* Tetraethylammonium chloride.

brain and also on account of the decreased flow to the viscera there is an increased supply to the limbs.

Electrocardiographic findings

These are remarkably mild. They are to be explained chiefly on the basis of the Valsalva effect, that is, an effect analogous to that which occurs in the cardiovascular system when one strains to breathe out against resistance. When an ECG is taken during the recovery period from a fit, the most frequently reported findings are (1) an increase in the size of the P-wave due to an enlargement of the right auricle which in turn is caused by the increase in venous return at the termination of the seizure; (2) alterations in the QRS voltage or of the R-wave, perhaps due to hyperventilation; (3) a change in the ST-wave may occur from the effects of the increased rate, anoxia and muscular exercise. These changes are similar to those noted in the Valsalva manoeuvre. Changes in the P-wave and QRS complex which have been reported are probably due to incomplete muscular relaxation. U-waves (which are considered pathological) have been reported in both unmodified and modified ECT. Some authors have reported an improvement in ECG patterns after ECT which had led to the presumption that some minor abnormalities, which were present before ECT, were psychogenic in origin. Arrhythmias are not uncommon after ECT, even when modified, but are less frequent if oxygen is employed. Atropine or quinidine, however, inhibits them. Beparon (tetraethylammonium chloride) is even more effective in this respect.

Respiration and blood chemistry

In an unmodified fit, apnoea occurs as soon as the current is switched on and persists until the tonic phase, when forced expiration ensues. This apnoea in expiration lasts 15 to 20 sec beyond the termination of the seizure. After that there is irregular and insufficient breathing. This is followed by a period of over-breathing which lasts for several minutes.

There is thus an increase of carbon dioxide and a fall in the oxygen level during the seizure, with a reversal of these findings in the period of over-breathing. The administration of oxygen before the fit causes a fall of oxygen saturation to only 80 per cent instead of to 57 per cent. In modified ECT, oxygen saturation falls only to 90 per cent with correct technique.

The study of Perrin (1961) shows that premedication with oxygen, atropine and scoline greatly protects the patient against vascular accidents. The pentothal is necessary to allay anxiety and to prevent muscular pain caused by the scoline. It also emphasises the value of beparon or some other hypopietic drug, in preventing a dangerous rise of blood pressure and cardiac irregularities of sympathetic origin. These findings have a special importance in the treatment of older patients.

An example of how this technique can effect a remission in old people of a distressing attack of melancholia is illustrated by a female patient of 76 who became depressed following a slight stroke affecting the right side of her face and her right arm. Imipramine at first did not benefit her but she stood up well to 4 ECT's after which she made an excellent recovery and the imipramine then maintained the effect of the ECT and the recovery was a lasting one.

Cerebral congestion and oedema

This was reported as a cause of death before the advent of scoline, but it generally occurred in patients who had some serious disease, or possibly who were for some reason over-sensitive to the electric stimulus. A fat embolus can result not only from a fracture of bone but from hypercholesteraemia. This can result from violent muscular contractions but should not occur if scoline is used. No patient has been reported to have died from a status epilepticus unless there were gross disease of the brain.

Respiratory complications

Deaths have occurred from pulmonary abscess. This suggests that the patient's mouth and throat should be free of infection before treatment is given; it should be remembered that the nose and sinuses are capable of holding as much as 100 ml of infected mucus or pus. Another possible accident without scoline is that the patient might bite so tightly on a tooth as to dislodge it so that it is sucked into the larynx and trachea. Cyanosis may suddenly occur immediately after the convulsion, if continuous oxygenation is not maintained. In this case the patient is usually in the supine position and his tongue has fallen back into his throat. He should at once be turned on his side and the neck extended. The best attitude for him is for his face to be looking slightly downwards so that the saliva will flow on to a piece of gauze. An airway should be kept in position.

Pulmonary oedema

This is generally attributed to feeble action of the heart. It is more likely to occur if the patient's chest does not move freely for a period of time. This could occur from scoline paralysis or in intensive ECT or electro-narcosis if the correct technique is not used. The patient becomes blue and coughs up frothy serous fluid. We have had two cases of this but both responded well to treatment. Pressure with the thumb on the carotid sinus can sometimes raise the blood pressure with beneficial results. In-travenous nikethamide is useful but atropine is contra-indicated. The patient should sit up in bed in an oxygen tent. The oedema may take some 12 hours to resolve.

Pulmonary embolism

As already mentioned the greatest care should be taken if a patient has phlebitis of the leg or for instance complicating middle ear disease. The use of scoline however will greatly diminish the chance of an accident occurring even where phlebitis already exists.

Impastato (1957) has suggested a simple test for bronchitic patients. He asks them to cough and if the patient goes on coughing and brings up an indefinite amount of sputum this is considered a contra-indication.

Endocrine system and viscera

One death occurred in England of a patient whose thyroid had been operated on. A small vein ruptured owing to the increase of venous pressure as there was no supporting tissue around it. The rise of venous pressure would not have occurred with scoline. Maclay mentions a patient dying from ECT who had a goitre that was probably toxic.

If scoline is not used, the contractions of the abdominal muscles can compress a dilated viscus such as the ileum so that it ruptures. A patient of

Epstein died of a ruptured liver. Another patient died of a hernia which occurred during ECT and which later became gangreous (Dunlop). In another case a woman's bladder ruptured as it had not been emptied before treatment (Cerulli). These cases are all quoted by Impastato (1957).

The treatment of elderly patients

Where there is a clinical indication for ECT in elderly patients, there are very few diseases which contra-indicate its use. We have successfully treated patients with the following illnesses: coronary thrombosis, cerebral thrombosis, pulmonary tuberculosis and glaucoma (here it is better to instil eserine first). Patients with arteriosclerosis can be treated, even where there is an increased danger of epilepsy, generally petit mal, occurring after the course of treatment. Osteoporosis comes perhaps the nearest to being a contra-indication and we have known a fracture to occur even when scoline was given. Patients on prolonged corticosteroid therapy may also be poor risks because of osteoporosis.

We had one patient who had an arthrodesis of the hip after an old war wound and to whom two psychiatrists had refused to give ECT for fear of breaking the leg. Scoline however completely paralysed the leg, enabling a successful course of ECT to be given, and the man continued at work in a high and responsible post for a further seven years instead of going into retirement.

One final point regarding the treatment of older patients, which cannot be emphasised enough, is that the operator should not ordinarily give the shock until he has seen the fibrillation, as in such cases it may take 60 sec or more for the scoline to take effect.

Complications of pre-medication

There is no doubt that psychiatrists did not co-operate sufficiently with anaesthetists when curare was first introduced. This drug was used for ECT by Bennett (1940) before it was introduced into surgery. It was not realised that oxygen must be given under pressure throughout the action of the curare. It was unfortunate that deaths from curare occurred at the very beginning, by ill-luck at two of the best run hospitals, one in England and one in America and these disasters caused a delay in the general acceptance of curare and even of the short acting relaxants like scoline.

In our clinic we used a form of curare from 1947 till 1951 but from the beginning of 1952 we began to use scoline and have used it over the last 10 years. We have had little difficulty with either drug and certainly our patients have been saved many distressing complications.

Pentothal can also be dangerous. Generally 250 to 300 mg are enough. Halton (1947) has pointed out that it is especially toxic to the heart in the presence of hypoxaemia and for this reason the patient should always be well oxygenated.

It is appropriate to end this chapter on the complications and side-effects of electroshock treatment with Impastato's remark that attention should be paid to any abnormal reaction to electroshock, including post-ictal confusion, as this may indicate organic disease of the brain or heart. Such a phenomenon may presage a fatal outcome in a later treatment.

References p. 100

CHAPTER 4

Electronarcosis and Electrical Anaesthesia

The application of electronarcosis as a method of treatment of the functional psychoses was a logical outcome of the use of electroconvulsive therapy. At the West London Hospital in the mid 1940's we were giving electroshock treatment to out-patients. As already mentioned we were attempting to increase the therapeutic effect while at the same time reducing the unpleasant side-effects. Electroplexy at that time had certain limitations. Some thought it inferior to insulin coma therapy in the treatment of schizophrenia. Others however had found that if the treatment was given more frequently and with a greater number of applications, then the successes in schizophrenia approached those reached in insulin coma therapy. We considered that the success of insulin coma depended more on quantitative than on qualitative factors. At that time as many as 40 to 60 insulin comas were being given whereas only perhaps 10 or 20 ECT's were given. Sargant and Slater (1954) advocated that 20 more comas be given to the schizophrenic patient even after the mental state had become normal. Another consideration was that the insulin coma might last up to an hour but the effect of ECT was much shorter. However, if concentrated ECT was given, the ensuing coma lasted for a considerable period, followed by a long sleep. We were therefore interested to hear that Van Harreveld and Wiersma, two neurophysiologists, had co-operated in California with psychiatrists in an effort to produce a safe form of coma therapy by means of an electrical current. Their apparatus included a device by which a constant current was delivered to the patient. Van Harreveld had been working on the problem of electrical anaesthesia for some years (Van Harreveld and Kok, 1934). Some interesting work had been done as early as 1890 in France by a scientist called d'Arsonval (cited by Gwathmey, 1914) who had been using high frequency currents. In 1902 Leduc caused a state of apparent anaesthesia in dogs by means of a circuit in which the cathode was applied to the forehead and the anode to the sacral region. His findings are discussed later in the section on electrical anaesthesia.

Later on Van Harreveld and Kok were able to show that the same results as were obtained by Leduc and his successors could be obtained by the application of an alternating current in man. With his collaborators he overcame the difficulty of the initial excitement by giving the patient a convulsion and applying the narcotising current when the patient recovered from the convulsion. The anaesthesia was prolonged for a period of some 7 min or longer.

Van Harreveld and his collaborators (Globus *et al.*, 1943) made thorough studies of the neurophysiology of this condition in animals and this made it possible for psychiatrists to use the procedure with safety (Frostig *et al.*, 1944). The routine procedure was to apply a current of about 250 mA to the skull with electrodes placed bitemporally a little higher than the level of the ears. This current was passed for a period of 30 sec. The passage of this high current for such a long time modified the clinical appearance of the fit.

In the method used by Cerletti a current of 1,200 mA was passed through the brain for the period of between 1/10 and 1 sec. There was often a latent period of up to 15 sec during which the impulse spread physiologically from the cortex to the mid-brain where a trigger centre initiated the self-continuing tonic-clonic convulsion. In electronarcosis however, the passage of the current stimulated the pyramidal tracts so that after an initial flexion of the limbs, there ensued a strong contraction in opisthotonus. Owing to the continued stimulation of the pyramidal tracts the usual clonic phase was masked. However the continuation of the current did not prevent respiration from reasserting itself about the 45th second. It was usual at this stage to reduce the current to zero and then within the next 30 sec to raise the current slowly to a value between 90 mA and 120 mA. This current was continued for about 7 minutes. The clinical signs which indicated that the patient was in the correct degree of narcosis were that his arms were flexed at the elbow in a state of hypertonus and that there was a slight stridor, although the patient could still breathe easily. If the patient became too "light" then the current was gradually increased in strength. Some workers used movable electrodes which could be slid one at a time along a rubber band encircling the patient's head. If the patient was too "deep" then one could move the electrodes forward and the respiration ceased to be embarrassed. On the other hand if the patient were getting too light one could move the electrodes back. We at the West London Hospital arranged for the construction of an apparatus which could produce a continuous current from the mains and which would have an ammeter, so that the intensity of the current could be measured throughout the treatment (Paterson, 1948 a).

We found that this technique was quite easy to apply and we used not only pentothal but also a form of curare. The patients whom we treated were generally those who were seen very early in the course of their psychosis as they were for the most part out-patients or in-patients in our general hospital. The recency of the psychosis and the good physique of most of the patients made the prognosis good. It was therefore a gratifying experience to be able to demonstrate a patient in a state of electronarcosis for some 12 or 15 min, at the end of which time the patient woke up and within a minute of waking was enjoying a cup of tea: within three hours he was able to carry on with his ordinary work. It was at once evident that this type of treatment was a great advance on electroshock. The therapeutic effect was certainly greater and we found that it was of especial use in distressing cases of chronic anxiety with panics which could not otherwise be effectively treated unless perhaps with continuous sleep. If one treated such cases with electroshock it generally took a concentrated course of treatment to get them well and there was apt to be a certain degree of mental confusion which however was hardly noticeable when they were treated with electronarcosis (Paterson, 1948 b and c).

The following points seemed to show that electronarcosis was superior to electroshock (Paterson and Milligan, 1947):

(1) It was more effective in cases of paranoia and of severe prolonged anxiety with panic;

(2) at that time we had a number of epileptics who came to the clinic because they might be going on holiday and wanted to have a convulsion on the day before their departure in order to obviate a fit at an inconvenient time; these were patients who were receiving the limit of anticonvulsant drugs; we found that if we gave electronarcosis, the period of freedom from fits was longer than with electroshock;

(3) Ellis and Wiersma (1945) had shown that there were marked changes in the functioning of the endocrine glands following electronarcosis and this was a pointer to the clinical effect being greater;

(4) the patients told us that they received a greater "lift" from the treatment. Van der Beek's (1953) monograph testified to the superiority of electronarcosis over electroshock.

Kalinowsky and Hoch (1961) state that the depressive patient requires as many electronarcosis treatments as he does electroshock treatments and that this allegedly shows that electronarcosis is no more effective. This is certainly not our experience. Those who have tried out electronarcosis over a considerable period however and who have studied the technique and the physiology of it, almost all agree that it is more effective than ECT. An exception was L. Rees (1949).

There have been some misunderstandings about electronarcosis which explain perhaps the prejudice which has existed about it. In the first place the Californian technique of passing a current throughout the convulsion has been thought by some to be a necessity for electronarcosis. In fact the best technique is simply to give an ECT in the ordinary way. It is better however to give a current which causes a considerable degree of stimulation of the cortex so that the patient becomes unconscious and has a strong fit. It would not be advisable to give a convulsion with the technique of brief stimulus therapy which produces a Jacksonian fit without immediate loss of consciousness.

There has recently been an interesting study by Cronholm and Ottosson (1960) in which they compared the effects of giving (i) a threshold convulsion, (ii) a threshold convulsion modified by an anti-convulsive drug, lignocaine B.P., (iii) a markedly supraliminal stimulation. The ultimate therapeutic effects of (i) and (iii) were somewhat similar although (iii) was accompanied by more memory disturbance; (ii) had less therapeutic effect. The conclusion drawn was that the convulsion was the essential therapeutic agent, and a threshold dose was indicated to prevent confusion. As is stated by Kalinowsky and Hoch (1961) future research must take this careful study into account. We would agree with this view, but we consider that the state of coma is important, e.g. whether there is electrical silence or merely slow waves, and whether as in electronarcosis the comatose state is prolonged. The relative therapeutic failure with lignocaine may be associated with the fact that the anti-convulsant drug almost eliminated the coma. On the whole supraliminal stimuli of moderate degree do not cause much memory disturbance. Schizophrenics treated by Thorpe and Baker (1958) with twenty ECT's were not affected psychologically to a worse degree than those subjected to insulin coma therapy.

The second misunderstanding about electronarcosis concerns the second phase, when a sub-convulsive current is passed through the brain. It has been argued that a sub-convulsive current has no therapeutic value. When for instance a patient has a petit-mal attack instead of a grand-mal during ECT, no benefit ensues. It has also been argued that sub-convulsive electrical stimulation has no value in the treatment of neuroses. In such cases the patient is given pentothal and it is thought that the drug, and not the electrical stimulation, may be responsible for any improvement that may occur. The fallacy of this is that in some techniques employed sub-convulsive electrical stimulation has been of such a feeble intensity that the current has not passed through the brain. As we have shown elsewhere, however, if a current is passed through the brain of sufficient strength to stimulate the sub-cortical centres, then an abreaction will occur of quite dramatic intensity. It can safely be said therefore that the sub-convulsive current which is passing through the brain in the second half of electronarcosis has a definite physiological effect. Its chief action however is to prolong the comatose state produced by the original convulsion. During this period there is pronounced activity of the autonomic nervous system, just as there is in the case of the insulin coma. It might be expected therefore that the current would have a therapeutic effect on the same principle that we have mentioned previously, viz., that a stressor can cause a reversal of symptoms in the case of a functional psychosis. We might add further that a more pronounced stress can produce a more radical and complete reversal.

A film made by us in 1947 showed what we considered to be the best technique for giving electronarcosis. We used pentothal, atropine and tubocurarine. Two psychiatrists who observed our methods wrote valuable papers on electronarcosis about that time. One was Monro (1950) whose paper on electronarcosis in schizophrenia was a model of what a clinical trial of this kind should be. He compared 152 cases of schizophrenia with a control group. Monro gave an adequate number of treatments, in some cases as many as 40. He found that a number of patients only showed improvement after as few as 10 treatments. The results he obtained were that there were 5 recoveries in the treated group for every 3 spontaneous recoveries. Furthermore the treated cases were in hospital only about half the time of the others, *i.e.* 15 weeks on an average instead of 28 weeks. He compared these results with those obtained by Malzberg (1938) for the New York State Hospitals, where the proportion of recoveries under insulin coma therapy for schizophrenia was only in the proportion of 4 to 3. Monro however was modest in his claims and said that there might be some relapses from these immediate results and that the paper did not militate against the claim that insulin coma was still the best treatment. It is strange that Kalinowsky and Hoch (1961) however quote Monro as advising strongly against further use of this treatment. Monro in fact found no ill effects from it and it would seem strange to condemn a treatment which halves the period of time which a patient spends in hospital and which increases the number of recoveries in the proportion of 5 to 3.

Monro's work is of theoretical importance because it shows that stress treatment administered to patients in a humane manner like that of electronarcosis, if given in sufficient amount, is extremely effective, even in patients who have been ill between 1 and 2 years. Monro in fact obtained a social remission in 20 per cent of his cases who had been ill between 1 and 2 years.

Harris (1950) described the effects of giving electronarcosis to 70 patients. In this series Harris was working with an anaesthetist. In this way he avoided the difficulties that were encountered by psychiatrists who had reported unfavourably on electronarcosis (e.g. Garmany and Early, 1948). These included burns, apnoea, apprehension on the part of the patient; waking up in the middle of the treatment in a state of fear. He used a modification of treatment which is of some interest—giving 200 mA throughout without lowering the current. The patient began to breathe at 45 seconds even though the current was continued. Harris wrote that the high current ensured that no patient would become conscious during the treatment. However he had cases of patients collapsing during treatment, which does not often occur with a lower current. Harris's paper does not support the thesis of Kalinowsky that electronarcosis is not better in cases of depression than is electroshock. Harris treated 32 cases of depression with electronarcosis of whom 19 had previously been treated unsuccessfully with ECT. Of the latter, 15 remitted with electronarcosis. Harris did not give as many treatments as Monro and for this reason perhaps his results with schizophrenia were not as impressive. Only 11 of 30 cases recovered or were considerably improved. Harris's patients preferred that treatment to electroshock. He found electronarcosis particularly valuable in severe chronic anxiety cases with panic, and also in paranoid states. The patients were surprisingly undisturbed throughout the whole course of treatment and were able to resume their usual activities within three hours. It had the added advantage that it could be given in cases of schizophrenia over the age of 40 where insulin coma was contra-indicated.

Soon after the advent of electronarcosis the muscle relaxant, known in Britain as scoline and in the U.S.A. as anectine, was used for ECT. This drug completely altered the character of ECT. It greatly increased the safety of the procedure so that even infirm patients could be treated. It could also be given in much more intense form without upsetting the patient. For this reason many psychiatrists were content to give ECT in concentrated form rather than give electronarcosis which is more time-consuming and involved a rather more difficult technique.

By 1952 ECT was being used more frequently in the treatment of schizophrenia and was given in a sufficient number of applications. We at that time were using electronarcosis. A valuable feature of the machine was that it measured the current which was passing through the patient's brain. When a physiologist is using electrical stimulation of the nervous system he thinks in terms of the intensity of the current and not in terms of the electrical energy applied. If the current can be set and monitored, and if it is kept constant despite changes in the resistance of the cranium, then the patient is not in danger of being subjected to too high an intensity. The electronarcosis machine is the safest for applying a current for ECT because it is then impossible to apply such a high current as to cause surgical shock, confusion or headache. It ensures that a liminal and not a supra-liminal current is used in each case.

Nowadays it is certainly of value for the psychiatrist to have as part of his armamentarium the facilities for giving electronarcosis to the occasional patient who is suffering from severe anxiety which does not yield to psychotherapy and where there are attacks of panic. The effects of electronarcosis can be much more rapid than treatment with sedatives. Sometimes, too, there are contra-indications to the prolonged use of sedatives. A machine of this kind can also be used for subconvulsive electrical stimulation.

In conclusion one can say that there is an alternative to the advice often given in textbooks that the psychiatrist should use as simple an apparatus as possible and give electroshock as infrequently as possible. This alternative is to use a machine which measures the current and not the voltage. The psychiatrist can then use not only ECT but also electronarcosis, as well as subconvulsive electrical stimulation. The last is used as a method of abreaction.

Electronarcosis: Notes on technique

Preparation of the patient is the same as for electroshock. The dose of atropine should not be less than 1/75 grain ($=$ 1 mg) because salivation is likely to be more marked than in ECT, especially if the electrodes are far back. The effect of 30 mg of scoline will last into the second phase when a lower current will be in use and when there will be no danger of a fracture.

The aim of the treatment is to keep the patient in a comatose state for a longer time than occurs with ECT. It is not necessary to use the original technique of maintaining a current of 200 to 300 mA for a period of 30 sec. An ordinary ECT ensures that the patient will go into a deep coma.

After the convulsion, the current is turned slowly up to a value between 90 and 140 mA. The patient thereafter lies in a flaccid state. The arms are flexed at the elbow. During that time the current can gradually be raised to a level where the patient shows a slight degree of stridor by the approximation of the vocal chords. The patient is thus able to breathe easily and we have never known a patient to wake up if the stimulation was sufficient to cause this stridor.

The patient should have been flooded with oxygen before the treatment began but it is not always necessary to continue it throughout the second stage. A nurse should have her finger on the pulse throughout the treatment. The pulse is not generally palpable for some seconds during the high current, though it may be if atropine and scoline are used, but if there is any subsequent feebleness or irregularity this should be reported at once.

It is better to begin with relatively short periods of narcosis and to increase the duration with each treatment. It is important to see that the patient breathes freely throughout the treatment. If there is much cyan-

References p. 100

osis or restricted movement, this predisposes to a serious complication, namely pulmonary oedema. Patients with a history of nephritis should not be given the treatment as in this case there would be a predisposition to pulmonary oedema.

Some workers have reported a sudden collapse of the patient in a condition resembling surgical shock. We have never seen this but the treatment indicated is to apply artificial respiration with oxygen under pressure and apply nikethamide and also to raise the foot of the bed.

Electrical anaesthesia and "electrical sleep"

The anaesthetists have helped to make ECT much more safe and effective. It is hoped that anaesthetists will help further to solve the problem of giving electronarcosis, or a similar technique in a more efficient manner than has pertained up to the present. This would be of interest to them, for the technique of electronarcosis as employed by psychiatrists is also a form of electric anaesthesia. In a typical instance the patient is insensitive during the second part of electronarcosis. One could pinch, cut, or pierce him with impunity. For surgical purposes, however, the two disadvantages of this method are that it requires a grand-mal convulsion at its beginning and that the muscles are in a state of hypertonus throughout the procedure. It would be more convenient if the narcosis could be generated without any initial excitement on the part of the patient and also if the muscles could be reduced to a hypotonic state. This problem has exercised the minds of the medical profession for a long time. For instance, on the 21st of July, 1902 the French Academy of Science was addressed by d'Arsonval who read a paper written by Stéphane Leduc (Leduc, 1902). He described how a large anode was put on the shaved sacrum of a dog and a small cathode on the forehead. Leduc used a unidirectional current of a frequency of between 150 and 200 cycles per second. He writes "The voltage is rapidly increased at the beginning until there is a production of generalised contractions. The animal falls on its side and respiration stops. We gradually lower the voltage until the respiration recommences. At a certain level we obtain a quiet and regular sleep. The respiration and pulse continue as before but all the functions of the brain are suppressed. The animal, whether it is a dog or a rabbit, remains lying down in a deep sleep. The muscles are completely hypotonic. The animal does not respond to being pinched or cut. Occasionally however there are some reflex movements. This state may last for 2 hours, without there being any alteration in the animal's health. The animal wakes up immediately, and after the treatment seems more active than previously. The current does not appear to be painful because there are no movements of defence or flight". Leduc writes further "If we raise the current slowly so as not to go above the necessary dosage, we have a brief period of clonic contraction and of restlessness analogous to that which is seen with chloroform anaesthesia. In that case it takes longer to obtain sleep, and the procedure appears to be more distressing. The animal usually voids the rectum and the bladder. The average current is between 2 and 10 mA." He sums up by saying that with currents of this kind he can obtain a complete inhibition of most of the centres in the brain without inflicting any pain on the animal, and leaving the respiratory and circulatory centres intact. In this way he obtains a quiet prolonged sleep and a complete general anaesthesia. The anaesthesia can be terminated at once and there are no unpleasant after-effects. He also points out that one can cause a temporary local anaesthesia by applying an electric current to a peripheral nerve.

The French were not slow to apply this method to the human subject. Leduc was the first to submit himself to electric sleep. Rouxeau and Malherbe applied the current; but the experiment was not pushed far enough to produce complete anaesthesia (Leduc *et al.*, 1902); 35 V and 4 mA were used centrally. Leduc was still conscious but could not move. He was anaesthetic. See Robinovitch, L. G. (1910) in "Anaesthesia", edited by Gwathmey, Appleton, New York, p. 633.

Leclerc (1910) describes two cases, one of whom, a woman with a large tumour, died after three-quarters of an hour. From his description the electronarcosis was just the same as that used by psychiatrists, in that it began with a convulsion and the muscles were in a state of hypertonia. This hypertonus is probably due to stimulation of the pyramidal tracts. The famous French surgeon Tuffier, working with Jardry, also used this method but soon gave it up.

Van Harreveld is probably the greatest authority on this subject. He and his colleagues made strength-frequency curves for patients at the same level of electronarcosis (Van Harreveld *et al.*, 1942). In this way he showed that a current of 60 cycles per second was quite feasible. He also demonstrated that alternating currents were just as good as any other type of stimulus for producing electronarcosis, and that the duration of stimulus with AC was suitable for this purpose. An American, Knutson (1954) met many difficulties in attempting to use electronarcosis for anaesthetic purposes. But Hardy *et al.* (1961) after 4 years' study of electrical anaesthesia in dogs felt that they had overcome these difficulties and could go on to use it in man. They reported two cases in which the initial discomfort of the passage of the current was successfully overcome by the administration of a short-acting barbiturate. The muscle movements were controlled by suxamethonium. Total myoneural block was not induced, and the return of spontaneous respiration was used as an indication that anaesthesia was becoming too light. Though salivation was pronounced, no cardiac arrhythmia, tachycardia, or hypertension was noted. Tracheal intubation and assisted pulmonary ventilation were thought necessary.

An Annotation in the Lancet (1961) says "If this work is confirmed, particularly if the return of spontaneous respiration in fact proves a reliable sign of imminent return of consciousness, electrical anaesthesia may prove clinically useful." Robinovitch wrote (1910) "We produce electric sleep in patients suffering from insomnia by applying to the forehead the negative electrode shaped to the forehead and the positive electrode to the palm of the right hand. The current is turned on slowly, generally some 5 min being taken to reach 0.75 mA. When this amount of current is reached, the patient feels a tingling sensation through his head and falls asleep within a few minutes. A small flag mounted on a little block of wood is placed on the patient's chest; the flag moves with the movements of the chest, and this is watched all the time whilst the patient is sleeping. The current is generally allowed to pass through the body for one hour, and is then turned off; but the patient continues to sleep for about half an hour. On awakening the patient feels refreshed; if he is very sensitive, he may remark that he feels a bit chilly. This feeling is probably caused by the vaso-constriction during the passage of the current." This technique, however, is probably without any significance for the psychiatrist at the present moment. It is similar to that employed by some Russians (Rokhlin, 1959). An account is also given of a Russian form of electronarcosis by Ananev *et al.* (1960). This writer however only describes experiments on animals and not the application of electro-anaesthesia to the human subject. He uses a combination of unidirectional pulse current with a galvanic current. This technique is not without danger as one animal died. An article by East German psychiatrists describes electric sleep in experimental animals by Kirtschev *et al.* (1960). In this case a current measured in microamps is used and the electrodes are placed one on the forehead and the other on the occiput. The frequency was 20 pulses per second and the average current was 50 to 100 microampères. It was claimed that this produced a well marked state of sleep in animals. The sleep comes on in most cases in a few minutes and lasts for 30 to 120 min. After the current is cut, the sleep persists for about another half hour. During electric sleep there is a lowering of the reactivity of the CNS.

Conclusion

With the classical method of employing electronarcosis as described by Frostig *et al.* In California in 1942 it may be possible to carry out a surgical operation. If the patient had his arms flexed and displayed a slight stridor from approximation of the vocal chords, one would conclude that he was sufficiently unconscious to be able to operate on him. The disadvantage would be that the muscles would still be hypertonic and the blood pressure considerably raised, possibly to about 230:150. These difficulties could however be circumvented by giving an appropriate drug to lower the blood pressure and furthermore by giving an intravenous drip with scoline. It is also possible that experimentation with the anode on the occiput and the cathode on the forehead might obviate some of the above difficulties.

It may be added that in America the petit-mal attack has been used as an anaesthetic Impastato (1956) induces in his patients a petit-mal attack so that they will not feel the pain of the muscular contractions caused by scoline. He prefers this to giving them pentothal which he considers dangerous. Further, pupils of W. Freeman who introduced the operation of transorbital leucotomy have used ECT as an anaesthetic. Immediately after the convulsion whilst the patient is still comatose, the two cuts are made and the operation is over before the patients wakes up. Kalinowsky (1959) also uses subshock as an anaesthetic for ECT.

References p. 100

CHAPTER 5

Subconvulsive Electrically Induced Abreactions

Neurophysiological considerations

In 1951 we realised that the clinical psychiatrist could not progress far if he continued to use rough and ready methods such as the use of the rather crude clinical machines designed for the administration of electro-shock or electronarcosis (Paterson, 1952 a).

We required a set-up in which electrical stimuli could be delivered to the subject in a way which would always be uniform and in which the stimuli could be varied in strength, duration, frequency, and in shape, as recorded on the oscilloscope. With the use of a polygraph to record physiological changes during stimulation (including the EEG) and a cinematographic film to record movements of muscles (often in slow motion), the whole investigation of electrocerebral treatment could be raised to a more scientific level. In addition, we were able to work with baboons, which are the most suitable animals for this type of investigation owing to their large head and general shape.

The goal of the neurophysiologist has been different from that of the psychiatrist. The latter has been in a hurry to achieve quick empirical results. The former has patiently devised experiments designed to show what the immediate effects of electrical stimulation on the brain actually are.

At the West London Hospital we have investigated what happens when a current is passed between two electrodes placed, let us say, 2 cm in front of and 2 cm above the ears. The current can stimulate three different types of nervous structure.

(a) Stimulation of the grey matter of the cortex This has sometimes been called indirect stimulation meaning indirect stimulation of motor tracts by way of contrast with direct stimulation of pyramidal tracts or peripheral nerves and it has the following qualities: (1) loss of consciousness if enough cortex is stimulated; (2) there is a delay before the corresponding muscle begins to contract; (3) if the cathode of a machine delivering a unidirectional current is placed at the upper end of the motor area and the anode 5 cm below and if the motor area is stimulated with a threshold current there is a characteristic smooth movement of the affected leg resembling that of voluntary movement; (4) the area affected is contralateral; (5) the number of muscles affected increases with the spread of the impulse over the motor area; (6) if the impulse is sufficiently strong, the contraction develops into a self-continuing Jacksonian fit.

(b) Stimulation of extra-cranial structures When the usual current is passed through the skull, usually with bi-temporally placed electrodes, the current spreads throughout the skull in such a way that only between 1 and 10 per cent of the current affects the brain itself. Among those structures which are also stimulated are the cranial nerves as they leave the skull. For instance, the V (trigeminal) nerve, when stimulated, causes contraction of the muscles of the jaw; the VII (facial) nerve, when stimulated, causes a "risus sardonicus" while the IX (glosso-pharyngeal) causes salivation. Stimulation of the X (vagus) nerve is responsible for many side-effects, including slowing of the heart and fall of blood pressure. The XI (accessory) nerve innervates the trapezius muscle. If the current is interrupted in such a way as to give ten effective stimuli or less per second then a clonus-like state is observed in the arms. The autonomic nerves are also directly stimulated, and at different stages of the treatment either the sympathetic or the parasympathetic effect may be dominant.

The direct stimulation described here differs from the indirect cortical stimulation described under (a) in the following ways: (1) it is elicited by a lower stimulus and so the patient always remains conscious while these contractions occur, (2) the contraction begins immediately after the application of the stimulus, (3) the muscles affected are on the same side as the stimulus—this is seen where a moderate unidirectional current is applied, the stimulus in that case being the cathode, (4) where there is a frequency of about ten effective stimuli or fewer per sec., the muscles contract synchronously with the stimulus, the so-called pseudo-clonus, (5) the current ceases with the end of stimulation.

(c) Stimulation of subcortical motor tracts The effect of this is similar to stimulation, just described, of the cranial nerves as they leave the skull,

in that there is no latent period; the effect is obtained with a lower current than that required for the cortex; there is "pseudo-clonus" with low frequency currents and the contractions cease at the end of the stimulation. It differs from stimulation of peripheral nerves, however, in that the effects are contralateral, because the site of stimulation is well above the decussation of the pyramidal tracts. If the stimulus is of moderate strength, summation occurs so that more and more nerve units are affected. If the stimulation is kept up the physiological spread of the current to the cortex occurs and from there it spreads to the trigger centre in the mid-brain so that a self-continuing tonic-clonic convulsion ensues.

Subconvulsive electrical stimulation

In 1950 the present writer had occasion to visit the Veterans Hospital, Lyons, New Jersey, and there he saw patients being treated by the passage of a subconvulsive electric current of relatively high intensity passing through the brain in order to produce an abreaction. The treatment was very dramatic. It was possible to see these men reliving terrifying experiences which they had undergone during the war and in some cases in civilian life. During the same visit to the States, however, one saw in other hospitals so-called subconvulsive electrical stimulation being given. But in these cases the current that was given did not appear to be sufficiently strong to penetrate the skull and affect the brain. The current might just as well have been applied to another part of the body. Many of the writings that appeared at that time concerning subconvulsive electrical stimulation showed that the writers knew very little about either electrical physics or neuro-physiology.

At the West London Hospital we had already constituted a team whose aim was to diminish as far as possible the ill effects of electric shock and similar treatments, and also to increase its therapeutic effect. This team now included a physiologist, Professor T. Gualtierotti. At that time there was very little co-operation between psychiatrists interested in neurophysiology and neurophysiologists interested in electrocerebral treatment. The gap between neurophysiology and clinical psychiatry is still unfortunately wide but it is likely to become less so if co-operation of this kind could be practised to a greater extent.

The clinical use of subconvulsive electrical stimulation

At the West London Hospital trial has been made of a number of different methods of employing abreaction in the treatment of patients who require something more than superficial psychotherapy and advice. This group includes patients with severe anxiety and with psychosomatic symptoms such as tachycardia, epigastric pain, asthma, stammer and the like.

The use of chemical abreaction has been largely due to the work of British psychiatrists, particularly Horsley (1936), Sargant and Shorvon (1945) and Palmer (1945) who have described in detail the emotional outbursts which can characterise the changeover from the neurotic reaction present to more normal adjustment. Nowadays the commonest agent is the combination of sodium amylobarbitone and methylamphetamine intravenously. This combination is definitely better than the use of each drug separately, though they have to be given at the same time from different syringes through the same needle. We have also tried out the administration of carbon dioxide inhalations. Though we have obtained interesting results from this method, we found that patients tended to be afraid of it. We have further made use of some of the new so-called psycholytic drugs including psilocybin. In our clinic we have made extensive use of hypnosis and hypnoanalysis, and abreaction frequently enters into this plan of treatment.

We did, however, find that the use of subconvulsive electrical stimulation had an effect which was different from any of the other methods, provided that the current applied was sufficient to penetrate the brain (Paterson and Conachy, 1952). There were two types of patient who were particularly difficult to treat by psychotherapy or otherwise. One was the war veteran who had been through distressing experiences and who presented a specific clinical picture. He was a man who had had a particularly well formed character and personality, and who had been subjected to a great deal of war stress. In civilian life he would be engaged in a routine job but would suffer from a perpetual feeling of tension and anxiety being particularly oversensitive to loud noises. He was also distressed because he could not experience the normal love of a father for his children and would also be irritable with his wife. Very often there was a feeling of pressure on the head or headache. The administration of

ECT in such a case was not generally successful. Nevertheless when sub-convulsive electrical stimulation (SCES) was applied, the patient would go into a state of somnambulance and relive some of the terrifying experiences he had undergone during the war. The reliving could last as long as an hour. In our experience the degree of disorientation and the vividness of the experience were more marked after this type of treatment than when abreaction by drugs was employed. There was a remarkable feeling of relief on the next day, and after several treatments this relief enabled the patient to benefit from psychotherapy and the end result was very good in many cases. The other type of case was one which would ordinarily have had a bad prognosis such as the aggressive psychopath who does not subject himself readily to discipline. Unexpectedly this type of patient was quite willing to have this treatment and in many cases he very soon went to the heart of the problem under the stress of the emotion generated.

Technique of treatment

About 0.5 g of thiopentone is given to a 10 stone man (63.5 kg) and the electrodes are placed just above and in front of the ears; if necessary a little hair can be cut. Nickel-plated electrodes are used with gauze well saturated with normal saline after the skin has been cleansed with "ether-meth" and after electrode jelly has been applied. Atropine 1/100 grain (0.675 mg) is advisable either subcutaneously or i.v. An airway should be used. (For dose thiopentone (pentothal) see also pp. 35 and 47.)

With the electrodes in position a current of between 60 and 100 mA AC is passed through the patient's skull. This causes a flexion of the arms at the elbow and of the legs at the knees. At the same time respiration is inhibited. If this current is maintained respiration will start again after a period of between 30 and 45 sec. If cyanosis is marked the current can be lowered at the end of 30 sec and then gently raised again. In some cases respiration recommences after about 10 sec with 60 mA AC. The flexion of the elbows and knees during the passage of the higher current is caused by stimulation of the motor tracts at the level of the internal capsule.

It may be remarked here that if the current is raised to 120 mA AC in nearly every case this has the effect of anaesthetising the patient and in some cases if this current is given for as long as 10 or 20 sec a convulsion may be caused by a spread of the excitation to a subcortical centre.

After 60 to 120 sec, if the current is about 60 mA AC the patient may raise a hand towards his head as if to remove the source of the unpleasant stimulus. When he does this, the operator gradually lowers the current. The patient may again raise his hand as the effect of the thiopentone wears of, when the current is again lowered. During this part of the treatment, the strength of the current is not sufficient to stimulate the diencephalon because the threshold is about 60 mA. The current however is tending to make the patient wake up and it is also stimulating autonomic structures outside the brain. The stimulation of the skin on both sides is also tending to cause some pain to the patient, who is just at or below the threshold of full consciousness. It is possible that this pain is a factor in causing the patient to show excessive emotion when he awakes; nevertheless we do not obtain as good therapeutic results if we do not initially give a current sufficient to stimulate the diencephalon itself. As the patient appears to be waking up, he is asked to squeeze the physician's hand and when he responds in this way the electrodes are removed. The whole treatment may last from 3 to 15 min.

In a typical case the patient remains in repose for up to half a minute, but soon begins to shiver and tremble, and there may be a marked sweating. Then he begins to weep or even becomes affected by convulsive sobbing. This may last as long as 20 min. During this time he may discuss at length some emotional conflict related to his maladjustment. In other cases the patient, though weeping, is unable to relate the affect to any particular subject. In still other cases the emotional release is not one of sobbing but of great excitement during which the subject relives some terrifying experience in the war. The patient may have described the event previously in an unemotional manner, but during the abreaction he may be unaware of his surroundings and relive the experience emotionally. In one case the patient, a British soldier, had been recaptured after escaping from a prisoner-of-war camp and had been thrown into a concentration camp. During his treatment eight years later he became wildly excited and threshed about with his arms in a fierce struggle with his supposed gaolers.

Other patients are in a euphoric state after the application of the current. They often express relief at being free from their haunting fears and discuss their symptoms and emotional problems fully. At this stage the patient often expresses gratitude that he can do this. He is in a highly suggestible state, a fact that can be utilised therapeutically.

The number of treatments varies according to the gravity of the symptoms and also to the nature of the abreaction. In some cases it may be carried out once only as an incident in the psychotherapeutic management of the case, while in others treatment may be repeated ten times, one being given every other day. With each treatment the violence of the abreaction tends to decrease. If the subject is an out-patient he can go home after an hour or so. The treatment is less disturbing than ECT and it appears to be without danger.

In this treatment, if an intravenous anaesthetic is used it is advisable to have a closed oxygen circuit with a rebreathing-bag, so that if there were any prolonged inhibition of respiration before or after the application of the electrodes artifical respiration could be applied.

Physical considerations

When the patient has been anaesthetised with thiopentone the current is raised to 60 or 80 mA AC. This appears to be about the threshold for stimulating the brain itself, for if electrodes are placed on the motor area, then there is a movement of a limb on the side contralateral to the negative electrode. With rather higher currents (about 90 mA) both arms and legs may be contracted by stimulation of the pyramidal tracts probably about the level of the internal capsule. If the current has a low frequency—for example, 10 effective beats per second—then the muscles are seen to jerk synchronously with the current pulse. If this stimulation is prolonged and the current spreads to the motor area of the cortex, then a fit may occur. With the level about 60 to 100 mA, however, the optimum results are obtained.

There is also stimulation of the autonomic nervous system, which in some cases is very pronounced. If atropine is injected before treatment, overaction of the vagus, which is stimulated on both sides as it leaves the skull, is diminished. Sometimes a sympathetic effect like dilatation of the pupils and quickening of the pulse is followed by vagal effects. More often, however, flushing and sweating of the skin are seen, as also are slight dilatation of the pupils and a rise followed by a slow fall of blood pressure, often reaching in time a subnormal level. A current of 60 mA will for a time inhibit respiration by approximation of the vocal cords from stimulation of the vagus. This effect is also lessened if atropine is given beforehand.

Although laughing and weeping occasionally occur when thiopentone is given alone without a current, these effects are brought out more frequently and more markedly by the addition of electrical stimulation.

Occasionally, after the early treatments, a patient complains of a certain degree of nausea, or of an increase of mental depression, or of a feeling of malaise lasting a day or so, although the last is very rare. As a rule, however, the relief of tension easily outweighs any transitory feeling of malaise.

Clinical material

One clinical series consisted of 50 (27 male and 23 female) relatively young subjects, 21 aged 20-28, 18 30-39, 7 40-49, 2 in their fifties, and 1 each in the subsequent two decades. In some cases only one treatment was given, but the most usual number was five. Two patients had 17 and a few 10 or over. The total number of treatments was 252.

Although on the whole relatively young, most patients had been ill for a long time: 43 (86 %) had been ill for over four years, 6 (12 %) for one to four years, and 1 for less than a year.

Special attention was paid to the question whether a terrifying experience has been a factor in the onset of the neurosis: 11 (22 %) had been subjected to one or more terrifying experiences in wartime, while 10 (20 %) had suffered a severe emotional trauma in civilian life. Attention was paid to whether the patient re-enacted the event with a release of emotion and whether the incident was in any way related to his current conflicts and symptoms.

The series included 15 patients (30 %) who had acquired abnormal sexual or other antisocial habits, some of a criminal character. In the ordinary way it is difficult for a psychiatrist to induce such patients to talk freely about their problems. If, however, at a comparatively early stage in treatment the patient could be induced to discuss his problems freely, there would be considerable saving of time.

On the whole the patients were emotionally tense individuals who complained of various psychosomatic symptoms, the commonest of which was the feeling of a weight on top of the head, or as if the head were held in a vice. Other symptoms in order of frequency were trembling feelings or "wobbly legs", over-sensitivity to sound, generalised weakness, indigestion, faintness and giddiness, ejaculation praecox and backache. More serious conversion symptoms were attacks of asthma or of severe epigastric pain without an ulcer, severe tachycardia, eczema, Raynaud's disease, writer's cramp and severe stutter. The actual clinical groupings are summarized in Table II.

TABLE II

Psychopathic behaviour disorders	10
Neurasthenics	4
Hysteria	17
Anxiety states	7
Obsessionals	7
Schizophrenics	4
Agitated melancholics	1

Three of those diagnosed as obsessionals had severe washing mania. Ten psychoneurotics with other diagnoses also complained of obsessional symptoms. Five psychotics were also included, four being schizophrenic and one an agitated melancholic.

Results of treatment

The characteristic effect of the treatment was to produce a highly emotional state of mind, most often weeping, so that the patient eventually became less tense and lost his psychosomatic symptoms. The most remarkable phenomenon was the manner in which patients talked freely about their personal conflicts. One patient who was shy and awkward with women spoke of his fears that his genitals were so small in size that he would be ashamed to marry. Case 2 (see below) lost his urge to interfere with young girls. Another man whose personality had greatly suffered from war strain had developed an urge to exhibit himself at a window, and this also cleared up.

Some patients used exaggerated language to express the relief experienced on the day following this treatment. One described it as "bliss" and another as "the happiest day of my life". It must be emphasised however, that the treatment was not necessarily curative in itself, but it permitted the psychiatrist to establish good rapport with the patient and to utilise this for subsequent therapy.

In a trial enquiry into fifty patients, thirty-eight (76 %) said that they felt at once a certain relief from the treatment. Only twenty-five (50 %) however, have shown a marked improvement since the treatment, lasting up to the date of writing, that is, from six months to two years. In some cases severe physical symptoms such as asthma, tachycardia, and severe epigastric pain cleared up. These were patients who had failed with other types of treatment.

Attention was paid to the problem of whether patients who had incurred a severe mental trauma either in wartime or in civilian life eventually did better than the others. There were, in fact, 11 cases in which terrifying war experiences had been an important aetiological factor. Nine of these re-enacted their traumatic experience, some of them in a trance-like state, as described above. In the whole group the abreaction took the form of weeping more often in women than in men (16 out of 23 women and 11 out of 27 men). Another reaction was euphoria, sometimes with laughter, while others showed rage. The reaction depended partly upon temperament and partly upon the original experience. The mode of reaction could be suggested to the patient. Thus a man who was weeping could be made to show aggression if appropriate noises were "heard off". Similarly, a man in a state of rage could sometimes be quietened by a gentle voice. There were 10 cases in which the trauma occurred in civilian life, such as sexual assault, or a sudden bereavement. The abreactions in these cases were not on the whole so violent.

All these patients were found to have current problems which were instrumental in prolonging an anxiety state which had started in the war. The treatment facilitated the subsequent resolution of these problems.

It was found that those cases which showed a strong abreaction had a better end-result than those who failed to react, although there were some notable exceptions to this rule. The following figures seem to indicate that a good abreaction to an emotional trauma was of good prognostic significance: the 21 best results in the whole group included 7 out of the 11 cases that had abreacted a wartime trauma; the 13 worst results were on the whole characterised by a poor emotional response and poor rapport.

Even in the cases of two schizophrenics who had failed with insulin-coma therapy this treatment was useful. One of these became much less tense and thereafter at least almost lost a severe stutter. In another case the diagnosis of a doubtful schizophrenia was confirmed only when the patient during this treatment expressed grandiose ideas that he was one of the great intellectuals of the age and fit to associate only with them. Cases which failed to respond included two schizophrenics, a mentally retarded patient and an alcoholic.

With regard to obsessional illness, there were three compulsive hand-washers. On one of these the treatment had no effect and he subsequently had a leucotomy. The second, who had a depressive background, reacted better to electronarcosis. In the third case, however, the patient, who had been ill for some years, gave up a practice of spending half an hour washing himself after micturition. He returned to work after an absence of many months. He had intensive psychotherapy as well. There were 15 others who had obsessional symptoms of less pronounced degree in a setting of anxiety with psychosomatic symptoms.

Of the nine patients who did best, four were classified as hysterics, four as psychopaths (two being homosexuals), and one as a chronic anxiety case. Four of these had obsessional symptoms—one being the washer mentioned above, one had a "going-back" mania, one was ruminative, and one was a claustrophobic with fears of being shot in the street.

Illustrative cases

The following two case histories indicate what results can follow the treatment: Case 1 illustrated how a patient may relive horrific experiences during the treatment, and case 2 shows the successful treatment of an aggressive egocentric psychopath who was a parasite on society and who could not give up the practice of interfering sexually with young girls.

Case 1 — A male clerk aged 30 was first seen on July 7, 1947. He had developed an anxiety state two years previously, with recurrent feelings of pressure on the head, giddiness, tremors and inability to concentrate. He could give no account of why the illness should have started at that time. No progress was made with the usual psycho-therapy during which he relived a terrifying experience in an air raid at Canterbury during the war. On this treatment he improved for a time, but a year later he appeared to be depressed and was given some treatments with electroshock with only transitory improvement. On July 7, 1951, he was given electrical stimulation, when the abreaction was more intense than that previously experienced. This time he expressed great feelings of guilt for the death of three young soldiers in the raid as they had been carrying out his orders at the time. On four subsequent occasions the same scene was relived and the incidents were discussed until finally he stated that he had lost his feelings of tension, pressure on the head, giddiness, etc. He was later able to carry out his work efficiently.

Case 2 — A man aged 36 had suffered from severe mental tension for some years, complaining of giddiness and inability to go out alone. He had no intention of under-taking steady work. He had hitherto been teaching pupils to play the piano, but attempted to behave indecently to one young girl. He had decided to become a pho-tographer, with vague ideas that he might photograph girls in the nude. He stated that he had been rejected for military service. He was first seen on February 21, 1951, as fits of depression had caused him to consider suicide. His wife stated that he was aggressive at home, and on one occasion had put his hands round her neck threatening to strangle her. She stated, however, that she was quite prepared to remain longer with him to give him a chance to have treatment. She stated that the patient's father had been killed in 1916 as a soldier, and that the patient had been brought up to be com-pletely self-centred. During the treatments with electro-stimulation he was able to show great emotion and achieve a close rapport with the psychiatrist. He was able to describe how between the ages of 14 and 16 he had regularly had coitus with his young sister, who was 10 at the beginning. Since then he had been obsessed with the idea of sexual intimacy with young girls. He also related how in the second world war, with his mother's co-operation, he had run away and lived in hiding to avoid conscription. In the course of treatment he was able to discuss how his emotional development had gone wrong. He was able to lose his narcissistic attitude and develop as a member of the community. By the end of six lengthy treatments at weekly intervals he was on good terms with his wife and had lost his severe feelings of tension. He has since obtained a promising position.

Discussion of subconvulsive electrical stimulation

From our experience with this treatment we came to the conclusion that a distinction must be drawn between the effect of passing a very low current such as 10 mA AC between the electrodes and those of a high current of 60 mA or more. In the former case there was merely stimulation of cranial nerves as they leave the skull; for instance excitation of the facial nerve can cause a twitching of the muscles of the face, the IX salivation, and the X a slowing of the heart and respiration, while the XI nerve could cause twitching of the muscles of the shoulder and upper arm on the ipsi-lateral side of the cathode. On the other hand the stronger current actually passes through the diencephalon, as judged by the fact that it excites the pyramidal tracts at the level of the internal capsule, so that the elbows and knees are flexed.

If a low current of only 10 mA AC is used, the patient may show excessive emotion when he awakes, but this effect may result only from the painful stimulus on the forehead. The same effect could doubtless be obtained by placement of the electrodes on many other equally sensitive parts of the body. The effect however has not in our experience the same therapeutic value as when one applies a current which is sufficiently strong initially to stimulate centres in the diencephalon. We obtained the best results only when we raised the current to this level.

This type of treatment is not widely used at the present time. There are several reasons for this: (1) it was peculiarly suited to war veterans and it was no accident therefore that the present writer's first impression of its efficacy were obtained when he visited a hospital for veterans of the second world war; (2) the technique does require a certain degree of experience and familiarity with manipulating an electrical machine. It also requires some knowledge of neurophysiology. However if a psychiatrist has read this Chapter, he is more likely to understand the significance of the various clinical phenomena which appear in the course of the treatment. If it is finally accepted in principle that electricity could be used to a greater extent for treating sexual psychopaths and psychoneurotic patients, then further research ought to be carried out into this type of treatment. This is already the case in Italy where to judge from the medical literature, a more varied selection of electrical treatments is employed. Certainly it was surprising to find that psychopathic patients for whom the prognosis is usually considered to be poor, reacted in a remarkably co-operative manner and the numbers which we treated have seemed to respond better than with the other types of treatment.

CHAPTER 6

Electrically Induced Cerebral Inhibition (Electrical Sleep)*

One of the most interesting developments of our investigations at the West London Hospital upon the effects of electrical stimulation of the brain, has been a study in which limited and specific areas of the brain were stimulated in such a way as to cause a generalised inhibition of the nervous system (electrical sleep). Our findings will be described in this chapter.

The physiologist with whom we co-operated and who designed the experiments recorded here was T. Gualtierotti, now adjoint Professor of Physiology at Milan, Italy. Gualtierotti had already observed that under certain circumstances a current passing through the brain did not spread but was restricted to the area directly between the electrodes. Since this observation might well be relevant to psychiatric treatment we decided to investigate the matter further. In the following account of these experiments any imperfections are entirely the responsibility of the present writer.

Technique for limiting the spread of the current to the area between the electrodes

The experiment was carried out on both animals (dog-faced baboons) and humans: (1) In each case a biological test was used to keep the strength of stimulation uniform for each experiment. The stimulus was between 1.5 and 2 times the threshold for stimulating the motor area as judged by the movement of a contralateral limb. (2) The electrical reactions of the cortex were continuously recorded with the technique

---

* The chief references in this Chapter are Paterson (1952 a), Gualtierotti and Paterson (1954, 1956) and Paterson (1958).

References p. 100

mentioned below. (3) The results were interpreted in the light of our knowledge of the physiology of the structures stimulated. A technique was used which prevented the spread of the current beyond a narrow line passing straight between the two electrodes. Square or sawtooth uni-directional pulses of 1.5 to 2 sigma duration at frequencies of from 4 to 250 per sec were used. Unpolarised silver chlorided electrodes about 7 mm in diameter were employed for stimulation and recording, the subject being earthed at the anode. With this technique there was no spread of the current at or near the threshold. A film showed the move-ment of the right fore-paw of a baboon and of a hand in man when the cathode was placed over the appropriate area of the motor cortex on the opposite side. A second method of demonstrating that the current is limited is by recording the electrical activity of the cortex during or immediately after stimulation. This was recorded through differential amplifiers with independent AC and DC control (Barron and Matthews, 1938), and a double beam cathode tube. A second record showed action potentials appearing over the stimulated point but not at a point located 1.5 cm posteriorally. This technique can therefore be used in areas of the brain other than the motor area. This recording of cortical potentials also demonstrates that such events as the peripheral contraction of a muscle is being caused by this particular cortical stimulus and not for instance by a direct stimulation of peripheral nerves or of pyramidal motor tracts.

Stimulation of an inhibitory (sleep) centre in the mid-brain in the baboon and in man

Having ascertained that it was possible to stimulate a limited area of the brain we proceeded further to investigate the problem of stimulating selectively, either the inhibitory (sleep) centre itself which is situated in the mid-brain immediately above the mammilary bodies on both sides of the aqueduct on the ventral aspect of the brain, or else part of an in-hibitory system connected with it. The part of the centre which inhibits the cerebral cortex lies anteriorly, immediately caudal to the diencephalon and perhaps occupying a small part of it. The nearest points from outside the skull to this centre are situated 1.5 cm above the temporal part of the zygomatic arch and 3.5 cm in front of the opening of the ear on each side. A line passing through the brain between these two points passes directly through the middle of the inhibitory centre. The line passes also through the middle of the temporal lobes in the lower half. Between the lobe and the inhibitory centre itself the pyramidal tracts are found lying in an confined space. It is for this reason that bi-temporal stimulation affecting the inhibitory centre causes a contraction of the muscles of the back and limbs.

To produce unconsciousness with a non-convulsive current, electrodes were placed bitemporally as described. Two main phenomena resulted: (1) a period of unconsciousness with average duration of 30 min (maximum 58 min) induced by a slight amount of pentothal; and (2) certain specific changes in the EEG. It was noted that the unconsciousness was produced by the minimum strength of current when the electrodes were in the position described. When they were gradually moved away, then a higher strength was necessary to produce the same result. A record demonstrated in a baboon after 5 sec bitemporal stimulation that action potentials were recorded close to the cathode but not from a recording electrode placed on the motor area 1.5 cm distant.

Unconsciousness therefore was the most striking effect of bitemporal stimulation. This procedure was applied to a group of 13 human subjects. These were patients who were being given electrical abreactive therapy as described already. These particular subjects however instead of being treated with the cruder clinical methods were subjected to the exact laboratory techniques as described above. A current which was twice the threshold necessary to stimulate the motor cortex was applied after the thiopentone anaesthesia through small silver-coated electrodes placed two centimeters above the temporal part of the zygomatic arch at the moment when the patient was beginning to recover from the thiopentone anaesthesia. The usual frequency was 250 pulses per sec. By way of control, subjects were given on other occasions stimuli at 30 per sec and on other occasions thiopentone alone. The results are summarised in Figs. 5 and 6. Fig. 5 shows the various durations of unconsciousness in the group of 13 patients and also two different patterns of reaction in two individuals in a number of these treatments. It will be seen that all patients except one remained unconscious from 20 to 58 min, the average duration being about half an hour. The degree of unconsciousness varied. In the deeper stages there was marked hypotonia in all muscles, reflexes were abolished and this corresponded to changes in electrical potential in the cortex (electrical silence). A careful watch was kept to see that respiration and pulse were not unduly inhibited and where this occurred the current was cut at once and artificial respiration applied. We consider that in our present state of knowledge there is some danger attached to this procedure

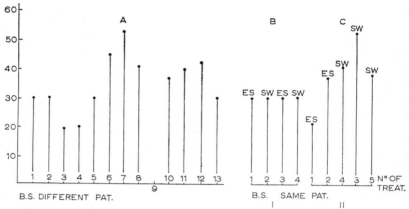

Fig. 5. Diagram showing the duration of unconsciousness in a group of 13 patients (A) and in a series of treatments in two patients (B and C). On the abscissa: serial number of each patient (A) or number of each consecutive treatment (B and C). On the ordinate: minutes of unconsciousness. E.S. = electrical silence. S.W. = slow waves. B.S. = bitemporal stimulation. This refers to the EEG recording immediately after the last burst: as shown, there is no difference in the duration of unconsciousness whether the EEG recording showed electrical silence or slow waves immediately after the treatment. (From Gualtierotti and Paterson, 1956; with permission of S. Karger, Basel/New York.)

unless the greatest care is taken to check the pulse and general muscle tone. In most cases however the subject's degree of unconsciousness was less than this and he would respond to stimuli such as hard pinching, which would cause unconscious movements, but no organised reaction was made to the environment. Only in the last 2 or 3 min of unconsciousness could medium or strong stimulation awake the patient. A series of treatments could provoke either a standard response, i.e. periods of unconsciousness of the same duration, as for instance in patient B of Fig. 5, or unconsciousness of different duration, as for instance in patient C of Fig. 5 and the one shown in Fig. 6. This diagram also shows the typical response of a single patient to 7 successive treatments (frequency 250 per sec) repeated every second day, to six bitemporal stimulations at a frequency of 30 per sec and to 5 treatments with the usual dose of thiopentone only. It will be seen that 250 per sec stimulation is able to prolong the period of unconsciousness produced by the thiopentone up to ten times, while

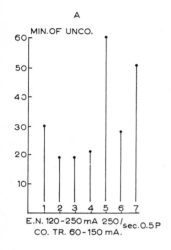

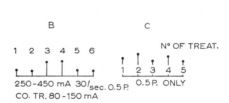

Fig. 6. Diagram showing the duration of unconsciousness in the same patient when the usual 250 per sec stimulation was used (A, seven treatments); the 30 per sec stimulation was used (B, six treatments), and pentothal only was given (C, five treatments). The amount of pentothal (0.5 P), the strength of the current corresponding to the cortical threshold (CO.TR.) and the one used for bitemporal stimulation (E.N.) are inscribed in the diagram. Abscissa and ordinate as in Fig. 5. (From Gualtierotti and Paterson, 1956; with permission of S. Karger, Basel/New York.)

stimulation at 30 per sec does not alter in any way the action of the drug, even when the strength of each stimulus is increased up to 3 times the cortical threshold. If a similar treatment is accorded to baboons for 5 sec without anaesthesia being given first, the same effect (lasting unconsciousness) is obtained with a pulse of 250 per sec but not with one of 30 per sec. (The exact threshold was not ascertained but is possibly about 50 per sec).

Changes in the EEG during and after stimulation of inhibitory centre

When a human subject was given an application of a current as described, with a frequency of 250 a sec, for half a minute, and this was repeated twice at intervals of half a minute, there was an abolition of all changes of cortical potential (electrical silence). Slow waves appeared 15 min after bitemporal stimulation and the EEG returned to normal in this case after 21 min. The fast activity reappeared just before the patient awoke. During the electrical silence there was marked hypotonia of the body musculature and absence of deep reflexes and this was followed by a rebound phenomenon of increased reflexes coincident with the resumption of fast activity in the EEG. There was no electrical indication of any sort of seizure at any time. These changes are different from those which appear during the action of thiopentone alone, in which case there are the typical slow waves but no abolition of fast activity. At the moment when the bitemporal stimulation is started the EEG has become almost normal, *i.e.* just at the moment when the effect of thiopentone begins to wear off. When 0.5 g of thiopentone is given, the EEG is normal after about 7 min. If three bursts of current are given to a patient when the anaesthesia is at its deepest, then the slow waves become much more reduced but do not disappear entirely. The superimposed fast activity does disappear completely. An EEG showing slow waves was obtained from a patient still unconscious 57 min after the stimulation. With thiopentone alone he would have awakened after 5-7 min.

Bitemporal stimulation of low frequency

The production of unconsciousness or the prolongation of unconsciousness produced by thiopentone anaesthesia was found to occur only with relatively high frequencies. We used frequencies of 200 to 250 per sec. Where however only 30 pulses per sec were used the following phenomena were observed. The spontaneous activity of the cortex was inhibited after each pulse but only for a fraction of a sec and after that a brief rebound increase of activity occurred. The record showed that the first stimulus did not alter the spontaneous activity; the second reduced it considerably, while the third almost completely abolished it. As this stimulation continued, the spontaneous activity was very much reduced but at the end of the application of the stimuli there was a rebound phenomenon and fast activity of increased amplitude was recorded.

Conclusion

The conclusion is therefore reached that the physiological effect of each stimulus is the same with the lower as with the higher frequency, but with the higher frequency the effect of each stimulus lasts beyond the beginning of the succeeding stimulus, and the effect of suppression of cortical activity, with unconsciousness lasts beyond the whole duration of the stimulation, even up to a period of 1 hour.

Another EEG phenomenon is that of the shift of the standing potential. It had formerly been suggested (Lloyd, 1941; Gualtierotti, 1952) that a shift in the standing potential towards the positive pole indicates a state of inhibition. In this case bitemporal stimulation with a frequency of 250 per sec causes the recording electrode situated over the motor area to become more positive in relation to the other. The most probable explanation is that there is a state of inhibition which has been produced by the stimulation of the inhibitory centre in the mid-brain. This shift tends to return to normal between the stimuli when a low frequency such as that of 30 per sec is used but continues throughout stimulation with the high frequency. The shift could be up to 3-4 mV.

Effect of bitemporal stimulation on the motor area

The following experiments were carried out on baboons. Three stimulating electrodes were used, one pair being situated bitemporally and the third on the midline on the upper end of the motor area. One could therefore either stimulate the upper end of the motor area by using as the cathode the electrode on the upper end of the motor area and as the anode the left temporal electrode, or one could stimulate the brain through the two electrodes placed bitemporally. The recording electrodes were placed as described below.

The motor cortex was stimulated by a current with a frequency of 4 pulses per sec and simultaneously a current was applied through the electrodes placed on the temples. The strength in each case was about twice that which when applied to the motor cortex just caused movement of a limb. The frequency of the bitemporal stimulation was 250 per sec.

The results obtained were consistent with the hypothesis that the bitemporal stimulation was exciting an inhibitory centre in the midbrain. The phenomena supporting this supposition were as follows:

(1) Immediately after the end of this simultaneous stimulation in the baboon lasting 5-30 sec, there was a bigger volley of action potentials following the first stimulus to the motor area.

References p. 100

(2) The second and later 4-per-second stimuli to the motor area for periods up to 10 minutes showed none of the action potentials which normally follow immediately after each stimulus of the motor area.

(3) After the onset of bitemporal stimulation, a positive spike followed each stimulus to the motor cortex, declining in amplitude after 9 or 10 stimuli but disappearing when action potentials returned. This was interpreted as a sign of inhibition originating from the stimulation of the inhibitory centre from bitemporal electrodes.

The results obtained with bitemporal stimulation did not appear to be caused by diminution of oxygen tension in the blood for in that case the EEG findings would have been different. There was no cessation of fast activity and there was a negative and not a positive shift in the standing potential. If the anoxia continued until a fall of blood pressure occurred, very large slow waves appeared with a frequency of 2 per sec, and all electrical activity disappeared. With bitemporal stimulation however there is not a fall but a rise in blood pressure if the strength of the current is above the threshold for the motor cortex.

Clinical application of the treatment

A headgear is prepared which consists of elastic bands which are sewn together in such a way that electrodes are fixed at the appropriate points. The electrodes are placed in such a way that there are two stimulating ones, one 3.5 cm in front of and 2 cm above each ear and one over the upper end of the motor area. The recording electrodes are about 2 cm in front of and behind this point. Little patches are cut out of the hair for the electrode placement. The skin is cleaned with ether and electrode jelly applied. The electrodes are silver coated and about 1.5 cm in diameter. The "helmet" is tightly applied. The resistance between the different stimulating electrodes is measured. This should always be less than 1,000 ohms. The patient then reclines on the bed and the EEG is tested. A note is made of the amount of alpha rhythm and the general appearance of the EEG. The patient is then given thiopentone and atropine. A test is then made of how much current is needed to move a hand or foot when the motor area is stimulated, and 60 per cent more of this strength is applied to the patient bitemporally. The reason for giving the thiopentone is that this test causes pain. The patient is given 3 bursts of 30 seconds each with intervals of half a minute between them. The EEG is recorded throughout.

The following is a protocol of such a treatment.

Case 1. Patient a man of 35

12.35   *p.m.* 0.5 g thiopentone i.v. and 0.6 mg of atropine

12.41½ *p.m.* Slow waves diminishing; some fast activity superimposed

12.42   *p.m.* 120 mA cortical threshold; patient given 200 mA bitemporal stimulation for 30 sec. Muscles remain tense throughout. Contraction of muscles throughout the body. Flexion of elbows; extension of thighs and knees; inversion of feet. Respiration inhibited from contraction of muscles. Half a minute intermission

12.43   *p.m.* Second burst for 30 sec. Again muscles tense. Again 30 sec intermission

12.44   *p.m.* Third burst. Musculature relaxes from stimulation of inhibitory centre. Excessive salivation requires suction apparatus

12.45½ *p.m.* EEG shows electrical silence

12.47½ *p.m.* Electrical silence still almost complete. A few slow waves

12.50   *p.m.* Slow waves increasing in size

1.18   *p.m.* Patient still sound asleep; does not respond to fairly strong stimuli

1.30   *p.m.* Ditto

1.45   *p.m.* Disappearance of slow waves and return of fast activity

1.46   *p.m.* Patient wakes up

The patient reported that a feeling of calm and relaxation lasted for over 2 days after the treatment. His symptoms had been those of extreme anxiety and suspicion. During the series of treatments the symptoms abated.

The following case however shows that there is some danger from the inhibition becoming too marked and affecting the vital centres. The treatment was carried out under laboratory conditions in such a way that the current could be cut at once if the pulse or respiration became inhibited and resuscitation could be given.

Case 2. Patient a man of 40

1.10 *p.m.* Given 0.7 g of thiopentone and 0.6 mg of atropine Square waves 250 per sec. Cortical threshold 150 mA. Strength of stimulating current 310 mA

1.11 *p.m.* First burst. After 12 seconds the patient's musculature became suddenly relaxed. Respiration inhibited. EEG showed complete electrical silence. Patient's respiration assisted and oxygen given

1.18 *p.m.* Some slow waves seen in EEG. Coughing and swallowing reflexes absent

References p. 100

1.32 *p.m.* Still asleep, breathing well
1.35 *p.m.* Still hypotonic and asleep
1.39 *p.m.* Still asleep
1.54 *p.m.* Awake. The patient then relived some terrifying war experiences while in a dissociated state
2.34 *p.m.* Still limp and half asleep but was soon able to give details of the experiences in the war which he related. Muscles still hypotonic. On physical examination patient showed nystagmus on looking to either side. There were persistent jerking movements of the eyes which were more marked when he focussed his gaze on some object. Past-pointing of left forefinger and left foot. Right side normal. Plantar reflexes flexor. Sensation normal. Felt some vertigo and headache. Loss of tone on left side. Pendulum movement of right leg below knee when jerk elicited
6.00 *p.m.* Neurological signs absent

Summary and conclusions

Hitherto psychiatrists have used electrical stimuli which excite most areas of the brain simultaneously. Such methods have been directed to causing a convulsion which leads to temporary exhaustion of the cerebral neurones. In the present study however a method has been described by which limited areas of the brain can be excited by electrodes placed on the surface of the scalp. The area which has been especially investigated is that which lies between two points on each side of the skull just in front of and above the external auditory meatus. The straight line which joins these two points passes through an inhibitory (sleep) centre, and stimulation of this area can cause a state of deep sleep in animals and in man. This procedure may however be dangerous for the patient unless precautions are taken to check the pulse and respiration throughout, and to cut the current at once if the pulse and respiration become inhibited, and if there is a generalised loss of tone in the skeletal muscles. The clinical effects of this type of treatment can be dramatic. The patient may sleep for a period of nearly an hour. He may feel very relaxed for a period of 3 days. Immediately after waking he may display intense emotion and either weep or laugh for a period up to half an hour. He may pass into a dissociated state in which he relives vividly a traumatic experience which has been instrumental in causing his illness. Serious symptoms such as auditory hallucinations present for some months or a washing mania may disappear after the treatment. One man who was cleansing his genitals 30 times a day gave up the habit permanently. He said "I feel that I have got back my aggressive attitude to life. I have got a grip on things again". He is still well and at work 10 years later.

There has not however up to the present time been an opportunity for applying this procedure to large numbers of patients. It is merely suggested here that this method of stimulating limited parts of the brain under controlled conditions may lead to a better understanding of cerebral mechanisms and to a higher degree of differentiation in the results achieved.

References p. 100

CHAPTER 7

Clinical Indications for Giving Electroshock

As already stated one may divide psychiatric illnesses roughly into three classes. (1) Organic disease of the brain, such as tumour. In this case surgical treatment might be indicated. (2) There are the less serious forms of psychoneurosis, and in the 1920's there was a great interest in the discovery that so-called "medical psychology" could elucidate and relieve these conditions by a "talking cure". (3) The functional psychoses (and we can include some severe psychoneuroses such as chronic obsessional illness in this group).

As we have seen, the third group does not yield to psychotherapy alone. The great discovery of the 1930's was that the application of stress through convulsions or comas could cause the symptoms to disappear in a high proportion of cases. The thesis is here put forward that these treatments in general were non-specific. The effects which they produced were not so much qualitatively different as quantitatively different. The reason why insulin coma was in some cases shown to be superior statistically to electroshock in the treatment of schizophrenia was that a far greater number of the former, in comparison with the latter, was given (*e.g.* Sakel advocated 40 or even 100 treatments). These were often given six days a week. Furthermore the actual stress lasted on each occasion a much longer time and the patient might be in a coma for as long as an hour. The patient underwent a good deal of suffering before he went into a coma. The death rate was much higher than in ECT and the side effects were much more serious. The advice to give only insulin and no other treatment to schizophrenics entailed only a small percentage being treated and that after a long wait.

Some writers have frequently ignored the dangers of insulin and constantly referred to the dangers of excessive ECT and to "patients' brains being battered by ECT". The fact is however that there is no evidence that ECT as usually given causes any damage to the brain whatever

(Globus *et al.*, 1943). The patient does not suffer much distress from having ECT and since 1952 when we began to use succinyl choline with pentothal, any danger to the patient has been practically eliminated. It is certainly more hazardous to cross a London street than to have ECT.

In ECT the stimulus (stressor) affects the brain directly and not indirectly and is thus perhaps more efficient. In assessing the different factors which have made the modern revolution in psychiatric treatment possible, Cook (1958) puts ECT first.

ECT in affective disorders

It is widely held that ECT is specific for depressive states. It would however be truer to say that depressions yield to a smaller number of treatments than any other syndrome. This applies especially to psychotic depressions. It is often said that the older the patient the better he responds but our figures show that patients in the 50's make the best recovery.

Psychotic depressions

In our discussion of the pathology of a psychotic depression, we suggested that there were three factors in the aetiology. (1) There is an innate predisposition to react to stress with a specific syndrome, *e.g.* shown by insomnia, anorexia, retardation and diminished spontaneous activity, or else by agitation, and subjectively by dwelling on unpleasant subjects, self-blame and inability to make decisions and by thoughts about death and selfdestruction; (2) the tendency to become affected in this way can be increased by acquired disease or injury; and (3) it can be precipitated by psychological factors, or viewed objectively, by wrong conditioning. Often, however, psychological precipitating factors such as frustration are not very apparent. As an example of the importance of psychological factors we may mention a patient with recurrent depression who did not have an attack all the time that he was a prisoner of war, although the cycle recurred on his return home.

When a patient is found to be suffering from psychotic depression, the question arises whether he should be given ECT or treated pharmacologically with one of the MAOI group or imipramine (tofranil). The arguments in favour of giving ECT are:

References p. 100

(1) The effects come on almost immediately. Indeed, it is claimed that ECT frequently prevents suicide (Moore, 1960). It can happen however that a patient commits suicide even after his first ECT. The reason for this is that the treatment has removed a certain degree of retardation and may have caused some degree of confusion. The latter is a dangerous symptom, as a patient is much more likely to commit suicide if he is a little confused than if he is clearheaded. Suicide however is very rare after ECT has started. On the other hand, the energizing effect of tofranil or a monoamine oxidase inhibitor may lead to a suicide. The euphoriant effect in this case comes on only considerably later (Arnold, 1960).

(2) One can predict almost with certainty that if 8 ECT's or so are given to a case of psychotic depression, the symptoms will disappear and the patient will stay well, especially if he is helped in his rehabilitation. This however is not true of some anti-depressant drugs. For this reason the term "neuroleptic" is inappropriate. They do not produce a chemical shock or stress to the patient of such a kind as to terminate the morbid reaction pattern. The drug merely interferes with the homeostasis or equilibrium of the morbid state and thus makes its continuance impossible: when the drug is withdrawn the morbid state returns.

Kalinowsky and Hoch (1961) state that if tofranil is given first and ECT second, the patient will require the same number of ECT's as usual, but if ECT is given first, much less tofranil is needed. This is not our experience. We have had cases of severe depression which did not respond to tofranil alone but which remitted when two or three ECT's were given in addition.

There is a belief held by some psychiatrists that patients show a phase at the beginning of their depression when they are resistant to ECT but that later in the illness they become susceptible to its influence. This type of case if it exists must be extremely rare. The belief stems possibly from a failure to appreciate the importance of concentrated ECT. I have had a number of cases of recurrent depression which have remitted after only six treatments with ECT. ECT definitely interferes with the rhythm. One man who for years had 3 months' depression twice a year with 3 months' freedom, after ECT has had a depression once a year, and it is terminated in 10 days by ECT. At the Cambridge Symposium on Depression 1959, Sargant indicated that the psychiatrist might hold his hand for perhaps 3 months in recurrent depression, as the patient is merely upset by it if he is in a "recalcitrant phase". He approved however of giving the patient perhaps 1 or 2 treatments a week when he is emerging from this refractory phase. Others at the same Symposium (1959), approved of this view, but one speaker pointed out that such views were equivalent to saying that ECT was quite useless in depression. One would be postponing the treatment until the patient was nearing recovery, but the patient who was nearing recovery was surely not in need of ECT.

Agitated depression

It is in this condition that ECT produces its most dramatic results. Although Cerletti had pointed out at the World Congress in 1950 that concentrated ECT was effective in agitated melancholia, it was remarkable how little this treatment was used in subsequent years. This was no doubt because the correct treatment was to give at least 2 treatments a day for the first 2 or 3 days, followed by daily treatment, which was followed in turn by treatment 2 or 3 times a week. It was this type of case which made such an impact on the morale of the staffs of mental hospitals when ECT was first used.

Tofranil is not always to be useful in agitated melancholia, even when combined with librium. Some psychiatrists use parnate combined with stelazine. It has been found useful to give an additional dose of stelazine at night in agitated patients in doses up to 3 or 5 mg as this counteracts a tendency to insomnia produced by the parnate (Milligan, personal communication). In our experience however ECT is preferable (see Oltman and Friedman, 1961).

Involutional depression

It is often said that this form of depression is the condition par excellence for which ECT is indicated.

With regard to very old patients, ECT is perhaps used less to-day than it was in the past and treatment with tofranil or fentazin may be tried first. Occasionally however one has a patient of advanced age who is chronically agitated and for whom life is not worth living. If the heart is strong enough to stand the strain, ECT given with scoline and pentothal can bring about an excellent result, and even in less successful cases it will have prepared the way for tofranil to take effect. Perhaps some geriatricians do not quite appreciate what psychiatry can do for old people. For example, a woman of 76 had a cerebral thrombosis with a right facial palsy from which she recovered. This episode was, however, followed by a change in behaviour. From being an energetic woman (she was a retired children's nurse who had been in one family for fifty years) who took a great interest in life, she became depressed, all day gazing into space and recovering only in the evening when she was relatively normal. A geriatrician was pessimistic as to whether psychiatric treatment would help. Yet four ECT's followed by a course of tofranil brought about a lasting remission from the melancholia despite the previous thrombosis.

Kalinowsky and Hoch (1961) pointed out that it is very difficult to treat successfully with ECT depressed patients with marked paranoid delusions. They state that 87 per cent of involutional melancholics recover with an average of ten ECT's but only forty-four per cent of the paranoid group, even though the latter have twice as many treatments. Nowadays however the combination of ECT with fentazin is likely to make the prognosis of this condition quite different, because fentazin has a euphoriant action and counteracts in a remarkable manner paranoid feelings in a large number of cases.

Post partum depression

A mild degree of this is not an uncommon complication of childbirth and cases of even moderate severity are often missed. Severer cases occur with a frequency of about 2 in a 1,000. It is extremely distressing for the patient in that she cannot experience normal maternal feeling for the child. We have known this illness to be the beginning of a rift between husband and wife that ended in divorce in more than one case. In the past the prognosis has been considered poor, especially if schizoid symptoms were added to those of depression. This illness if untreated may take years to recover completely. It is however responsive to ECT even if a greater number of applications than usual is necessary.

Jacobs (1943) pointed out that results with ECT in this type of case were satisfactory.

Seager (1959) describes forty-two patients with post-partum illness and compared them with women who show similar symptoms except that they are not puerperal, and also with puerperal women who are non-psychiatric cases. The women suffering from post-partum illness had more psychiatric illness in their personal and family histories than the normal puerperals but did not differ significantly from the non-puerperal psychotics. Seager thinks that the puerperal changes act as a stressor precipitating the psychosis. No detailed account is given of the treatment except to say that electroplexy, insulin coma and neuroleptic drugs were given as seemed indicated. The puerperal depressives and schizophrenics had the same prognosis as in non-puerperal cases.

Psychoneurotic depression

Such patients differ from the foregoing in that there is often a more obvious environmental cause for their illness. They may not fall asleep easily, but they do not wake early. They are not suicidal, and autonomic symptoms are not so prominent. Although good results are often obtained in this group with ECT, the percentage of cures is not as high as with the psychotic depressions. In our experience these psychoneurotic depressions often yield more readily to treatment with librium or phenelzine or both together. Sometimes however, a depression caused by a bereavement has been excessive and has cleared up only when ECT was given. The treatment of this condition is discussed further in Part II. Garmany (1958) finds ECT beneficial in many cases.

Treatment of mania

At the present time perhaps most psychiatrists would employ by preference a sedative drug such as a phenothiazine for this condition. Oles (1960) uses haloperidol for mania — and states that the drug is effective within a few days. The patient shows signs of Parkinsonism in about 80 per cent of cases. This is probably a better drug for mania than the phenothiazines. Sometimes however failures do occur with tranquillizing drugs and in such cases the application of two ECT's a day for three days followed by one a day will probably make a patient symptom-free in under a week. Lithium which is specific has been used in this condition with soms success. The carbonate is probably the safest form to use. Generally 250 mg thrice daily is sufficient, though twice this dose may be used (Noack and Trautner, 1951).

As the drug is cumulative it should be omitted on one day in seven. The patient should be symptom-free within two weeks. It should not be given to outpatients in large doses.

References p. 100

Chronic melancholia

Even with the chronic melancholic patient whose symptoms have proved to be more intractable than in the cases above, ECT can be a most valuable aid in bringing about a more satisfactory level of adjustment: Cook (1958) described wards in a mental hospital before the advent of ECT which were full of chronic melancholic patients such as are seldom seen nowadays. He also described agitated and violent melancholics whose symptoms abated when they were given this treatment. It does seem therefore that the freedom from symptoms effected by electrical treatment has made it possible in melancholia as in schizophrenia for intensive rehabilitation and occupational therapy to be carried out so that the patient can live at a more effective level. In this way he is a much happier and saner individual than his counterpart of thirty years ago.

Preventive ECT

An effective prophylactic measure is that of giving ECT before the next attack is expected in those cases where there is a regular cycle of depression or mania. This was first suggested by Geoghegan and Stevenson (1949). We have found that this procedure is often successful, especially if great care is taken to make the patient's subsequent environment as free from stress as possible. One of our female patients had a recurrent attack of melancholia every six months which lasted for about the same period. There were also some obsessional symptoms. This recurrent illness was present for six years before electroshock was introduced. She was given concentrated electroshock, *viz.*, one a day for five days at the beginning of the melancholia followed by an electroshock every other day until she had twelve in all, followed by two more at four-day intervals. This resulted in a remission of symptoms which returned to about half their usual strength and she was able to carry on with her work throughout the depression for the first time. This procedure was repeated on three occasions with similar results but later she was given one ECT a month for three months before the depression was expected and then four during the fortnight before it was expected. This procedure was much more effective than giving the treatment at the time of the depression. The patient's symptoms were then not serious enough to interfere with her work. At times they were absent and at their worst still tolerable. There-

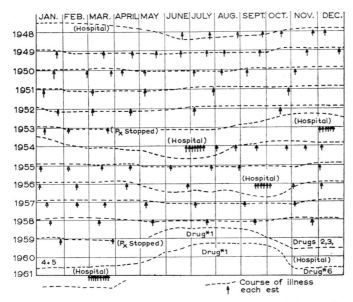

Fig. 7. Chart shows relation between course of illness and "Prophylactic Electroshock" (by courtesy of the *American Journal of Psychiatry*).

after the patient for ten years was almost symptom free. She had attacks which lasted two or three weeks instead of six months and only on one occasion did she need four ECT's to recover. She is no longer considered an invalid but is a cheerful individual who enjoys life.

The accompanying chart is from Hastings (1961). The patient had recurrent attacks of mania and melancholia, as shown. However the administration of one ECT a month as a prophylactic inhibited further psychotic attacks, but the patient unfortunately developed a fear of the treatments. He was therefore treated with marsilid for his depression but without effect. This drug is dangerous and has since been withdrawn from the U.S. market. He was then treated for mania by administration of thioridazine (melleril, mellaril) but this had no good effect. Only when he resumed his monthly ETC did he once more avoid the occurrence of mania and melancholia.

References p. 100

ECT in schizophrenia

At the Paris conference in 1950 Cerletti described the results of twelve years of treatment with ECT. He mentioned its efficacy in both depression and mania but he had been disappointed with the results in the hebephrenic form of schizophrenia. He realised however that it was effective in some other schizophrenic conditions. He observed that many more ECT's were necessary than in cyclothymia and mentioned twenty treatments as a reasonable number. He pointed out that ECT was an excellent treatment if the patient was seen early in the condition. He recommended concentrated electric treatment at that stage in order as he said to "block the onset of schizophrenia".

It is of interest that Robertson discussing the prevention of insanity in 1926, said there were two stages in the onset of a psychosis, (1) an initial stage when it was theoretically reversible, "when anything is possible", and (2) a later stage when there was definite insanity, the form of which remained fixed. Many workers have confirmed that this "blockage" resulting from ECT, often in concentrated form, causes the more florid symptoms to disappear and even the disease process itself. The diagrams from Blair and Brady and from Danziger and Kindwall (Fig. 4 on p. 23 and Fig. 2 on p. 22) indicate how effective ECT can be in early cases.

As already mentioned, however, Sakel was wise enough to advocate deep comas, long comas and frequent comas, and this quantitative difference tipped the statistics just in favour of insulin in many reports. Where the technique of electrocerebral treatment was improved and electronarcosis was given in sufficient quantity as in the report of Monro (1950), the statistics favoured electricity over insulin. It was surprising that in England the textbooks came out strongly in favour of insulin, for the younger psychiatrists still continued to use ECT with success; (Barker and Baker, 1959; Bourne, 1953). Norton (1961) shows that at Cook's hospital insulin declined in favour, and schizophrenics were hardly given coma treatment after 1952. Only about 1956 did ECT give way to some extent to treatment with chlorpromazine.

Many facts bear out the supposition that success depends on giving an adequate number of treatments. Before the advent of succinyl choline, electronarcosis was the best method of giving a more concentrated form of electrocerebral treatment and nearly every worker who tried it out thoroughly, reported that it was superior to ECT. The most favourable reports of ECT in early schizophrenia are from Italy where, following Bini's example, adequate courses are given. In the U.S.A. Danziger and Kindwall generally gave twenty to forty ECT's to schizophrenics, though they stopped when the remission occured. They showed that many more remissions occurred if forty treatments were given compared with twenty (Fig. 2). Some workers while acknowledging that ultra-intensive ECT can produce good effects without subsequent mental deterioration, state that similar results can be obtained by giving the same number of treatments at longer intervals apart.

Kalinowsky and Worthing (1943) have found that 68.3 per cent of schizophrenics recover sufficiently to return home if they are treated with ECT within six months of the onset of the illness. This compares with 69.7 per cent quoted by Cook for cardiazol. In New York State Hospitals, the corresponding figures in studies of ECT and cardiazol were 80.4 and 84.3 per cent respectively (Zeifert, 1941). Bockoven et al. (1951) have demonstrated the striking increase in discharges from mental hospitals since the use of biological therapies particularly the easily applicable electroshock therapy. As has often been stated, it has been this which had made the new humanistic approach to psychiatry possible.

A modern plan for the treatment of schizophrenia

In a recent study by Arnold and Hoff (1961), a view of schizophrenia is put forward, similar to that which has been outlined in this book. The authors believe that there is an inborn predisposition on the part of the patient to develop this particular psychosis. They believe that the somatic basis consists of "enzyme bottle-necks" in certain parts of the brain. They also think that stress either of a physical or of a psychological (environmental) character can trigger off the disease process. This reaction pattern of the patient may be in the nature of a retreat from the world (schizophrenia) or a "flight into reality" (mania). The patient's previous conditioning will also affect the nature of the inborn reaction pattern. They believe that the enzymic abnormality amounts to a "lesion" and that this causes a difficulty in the patient reacting normally to the environment. They maintain that shock treatment does counteract these enzymic deficiencies. After the patient has become symptom-free through shock treatment they emphasise the necessity for a prolonged effort at rehabilitation including the counselling of other members of the patient's family.

They have four treatment schemes for schizophrenia. One is ECT which is used in retarded and stuporose patients, where there is not much autism but only a mild thought disorder with fleeting hallucinations, generally of a visual character. In such cases there is an element of depression and so it is designated a "mixed psychosis".

Secondly they use ECT plus a phenothiazine in early schizophrenia where a remission might be expected. In this type of patient there may again be stupor and thought blocking with some auditory hallucinations. The thought disturbances are only of moderate degree and there are no marked delusions.

Thirdly they use insulin coma for schizophrenia where a successive attack is worse than a previous one which has remitted. In this case the patient feels depersonalised and thinks that he is being influenced from a distance. He has auditory hallucinations, often of a threatening character. It is interesting that they consider it worthwhile giving insulin coma to a patient whose illness is already of some duration.

The fourth type of treatment is the use of majeptil (thioproperazine). This is given for what is called a "process psychosis". This is where the illness develops gradually as in hebephrenia. The patient feels there is a hidden meaning behind innocent acts on the part of his neighbours; ideas of reference are marked; he has bizarre emotions, his delusions may become systematised for a time but later disintegrate, and much of his behaviour is shameless. He has no insight. Majeptil has the effect of producing a Parkinsonian state with torsion spasms in the patient. He remains in this state for some five days and if the spasms are painful or distressing he is given an injection of 10 mg of methedrine i.v. The patient is then rested for two to four weeks and the treatment may be repeated six times in all.

Arnold believes that the articifial production of a Parkinsonian state acts much in the same way as a shock treatment. Parkinsonism occurring naturally is generally characterised by an attitude of "indifference" which was the description first given to the effect of largactil by Laborit (see also p. 109). It would seem that the effect of majeptil in this respect is stronger than that of chlorpromazine.

These authors evidently realise that physical therapies must be thorough-going. For ECT they use atropine, succinyl choline and an i.v. barbiturate and they give three to five treatments in the first week, three in the second, and two in the third. The psychotropic drug they use is chlorothioxanthene (truxal, taractan) in doses of 150 to 400 mg in twenty-four hours and this is given before and after ECT.

They treat catatonia by giving six ECT's on the first day (three at a time on two occasions with fifteen minutes between the applications and forty-five minutes between the two sets of treatments). They give two on the second day, two on the third day, and one on the fourth and fifth day. The sixth day is a rest day. On the seventh there is one ECT, in the second week only three, and in the third week two. No neuroleptics are given whilst the patient is having ECT. This finding is in line with our own experience that concentrated electrical treatment is the best therapy for catatonic stupor. Mitchell (1952) described concentrated ECT as an effective treatment for prolonged stupor.

Lopez Ibor at the World Congress (1950) mentions that convulsive therapy offers the sole possibility of saving severe cases of catatonic stupor, while insulin coma can be very dangerous. He emphasised that concentrated treatment was necessary, as many as three a day for the first few days. Paterson (1952b) describes a catatonic woman of 51 who was in a state of terror from hearing accusing voices and who made a suicidal attempt, before lapsing into a state of stupor. She had twenty-three treatments with electronarcosis, twelve of which were on successive days. Considerable care was taken with rehabilitation after the illness. She made a complete recovery and was reported as completely normal ten years after her illness.

Arnold and Hoff (1961) are equally thorough in giving insulin coma treatment. They eventually induce comas lasting for as long as an hour and they are given six days a week. Between fifty and one hundred and fifty comas are given. If after twenty comas the patient does not show definite improvement he has a leptazol (cardiazol) shock twice a week after a coma. Great care is taken to educate the patient's family and to effect a permanent rehabilitation.

The figure quoted for full and social remissions for untreated cases is 40 per cent. With the above treatments however 85.5 per cent obtained full or social remissions, full remissions being 38.9 per cent for 118 cases in 1958-1959 as against 14.3 per cent for the untreated cases, which were 467 in number.

The figures for insulin coma in the years 1952-1953 (173 cases) were 46.8 per cent for full recovery and 80.3 per cent when social remissions were included. There were three deaths from insulin treatment. The authors attribute the fact that the insulin coma cases showed a higher remission rate to the finding that in time social remissions tend to become full remissions, as Achte also found in Finland.

These figures from Vienna contradict the opinion of Hoch (Arieti, 1959) in that the results from insulin coma treatment fall off, so that after five years there is no difference between the numbers of spontaneous remissions and remissions in insulin treated patients. These figures indicate also that the combination of active biological treatment with psychotherapy and rehabilitation can double the number of remissions when compared with an untreated series of cases. It has even been said that ECT is as effective as any other shock treatment if it is given early enough and with a sufficient number of applications, up to twenty or more.

In the paranoid form of schizophrenia, the phenothiazines have an almost specific effect, particularly fentazin which often substitutes a feeling of well being and confidence for a feeling of suspicion. We have seen many cases of paranoia which yielded to ECT or electronarcosis. Both Medlicott (1947) and Van der Beek (1953) had good results with electronarcosis in that condition.

Blair and Brady (1958) believe that chlorpromazine is much more effective in patients who have already been treated with ECT. They use a stepping-up process in which the patient is put on 300 mg of chlorpromazine daily for 8 weeks: the dose is then doubled and continued for four weeks, after which it goes up to 900 mg a day, and after a further four weeks, up to 1200 mg a day. This might be continued for about ten weeks, after which the dose is diminished over a period of a fortnight to 300 mg a day which is the maintenance dose. If the patient fails to make progress at any stage in the chlorpromazine treatment he is given a series of some six ECT's before treatment is resumed.

It would appear therefore that the modern treatment of schizophrenia by the phenothiazines can be improved by combination with ECT.

Conclusion

*The present status and future possibilities
of electrocerebral treatment*

Twenty-three years have passed since electroshock was first used by
Cerletti and Bini in Rome. At that time its chief rivals were cardiazol
treatment and insulin coma. There were also psychiatrists who had more
faith in psychoanalysis while others used continuous sleep or leucotomy
excessively. At that time ECT had the advantage over cardiazol in that
it was easier to give and that the patient became immediately unconscious.
Despite these advantages it was unpopular with psychiatrists. It was dis-
tasteful to witness; it was a crude procedure; there were many dangers
attached to it and it was described as being "empirical". It was difficult
to give any account of the rationale of the treatment (Sargant and Slater,
1954).

In the 1940's many psychiatrists were by temperament more interested
in the problems of psychopathology or in social psychiatry. If ECT were
to be a valuable treatment, the practising psychiatrist would at that time
require to learn all about anaesthetics and neurophysiology, and to be an
active clinician giving physical treatments. It was not surprising that
some rationalisation was employed to belittle the treatment or to shrug it
off as one of those fashions in medicine that would soon disappear.

Nevertheless since its inception in 1938 ECT was increasingly employed until 1953, when the neuroleptic drugs were beginning to be more
widely used. Cerletti has not been very proud of his brain-child, describing
it as a crude procedure which would soon be replaced by biochemical
treatments. At the Paris Conference (1950) however its indications were
described as being much wider than merely for depression alone, especially if it were given in more concentrated form or with a greater number
of applications. By 1952 scoline was being used and this gave a great

impetus to the treatment. The indications were still further widened, and old and infirm patients could be more safely treated. It also became easier to give concentrated treatments and for this reason electronarcosis, which was being used by many workers in place of concentrated ECT was employed more sparingly.

The popularity of ECT increased steadily until the advent of neuroleptic drugs. However recently a number of observers have reported that its popularity has again been revived and Holt in America (1959) and Curran in London (1962) have said that its use is once again on the upgrade. At St. George's Hospital it is being used almost as much as before the advent of neuroleptic drugs. Its chief advantages are: It is not hard on the patient, who is unconscious during the application of the stress. It is easy and safe to give and there are no ill effects except a transitory loss of memory, which with care can be negligible. It can be given to outpatients and it can be applied very early in the mental disorder. It does not negate the use of other treatments but on the contrary is synergic with insulin coma in schizophrenia. One psychiatrist at a teaching hospital reported recently that his colleagues in other branches of medicine were convinced that ECT was the only treatment in psychiatry that was consistently effective. It can be used as Blair and Brady (1958) have shown, in conjunction with the phenothiazines in schizophrenia. Baker *et al.* (1960) prefer it without phenothiazines. In comparison with the antidepressive drugs it has certain advantages. One can predict that with a given number of treatments the patient will make a lasting recovery: the results are obtained rapidly. With the antidepressive drugs however, the beneficial action is obtained after a greater period of delay, and recovery is less certain.

On the other hand in 1952 when the neuroleptic drugs were introduced, the climate of opinion was favourable to their reception. Many psychiatrists were dissatisfied with the methods of psychotherapy, and many recognised the limitations of ECT as used at that time. Objections were repeatedly raised that it was crude and empirical. It was hoped that further research in pharmacotherapy would reveal that the drugs had a greater degree of precision in their effect. The aim was to produce drugs which would have a much more differentiated effect on the patient's feeling and behaviour. Many psychiatrists who had belittled electroshock were pleased that psychiatry would now be more in line with the traditions of general medicine. Nevertheless, the hopes placed in the anti-depressive drugs, except in certain classes of patients, have so far not been realised, and for that reason the use of electrocerebral treatment is again on the up-grade. Fur her, the new drug "indoklon" has not been found so convenient as ECT as a convulsant (Impastato, 1961).

At the time when the neuroleptic drugs were introduced ECT was being given by junior Registrars (trainee specialists) working often alone and with no instruction from textbooks on the effects of electric stimuli on the brain and other organs of the body. The official textbooks advised that as little treatment be given as possible and retarded melancholia was almost the only indication. It was advised that only a small simple fool-proof machine be used.

Nowadays however because of the advent of new muscle relaxants, the indications for treatment are much wider. ECT has become respect-able by comparison with the neuroleptic drugs. Moreover instead of a solitary Registrar desiring a simple shock machine, we have skilled anaes-thetists interested in more elaborate electric machines which can give electric coma, electric anaesthesia and generalised electrical inhibition as well. It is because of this that full accounts have been given of these procedures. It is likely therefore in the future that if as much co-operation takes place between physicists, neurophysiologists, anaesthetists and psy-chiatrists, we shall see much greater advances in the treatment of mental disorders than have occurred so far. Up till now most University centres have concentrated on psychology and sociology. For the study of mental disorders however this is not enough. Electricity and electronics must be employed to study the working of the brain, the cortex and sub-cortex in disease as well as in health. The possibilities of important advances are great. So far, from the practical standpoint, we have found that elec-trically produced convulsions and comas reverse many psychotic pro-cesses without injuring the patient and that there are further thera-peutic possibilities in electrically induced abreaction, in electric sleep (inhibition) and electric anaesthesia. There is a great need at the present time for more laboratories where these subjects can be studied in con-junction with electro-encephalography, and with conditioned reflex tech-niques.

References p. 100

References to Part I

ACHTE, K. A. (1961), Der Verlauf der Schizophrenien und der Schizophreniformen Psychosen, *Acta psychiat. scand.*, Suppl. 155.

ALEXANDER, L. (1961 a), *Effects of psychotropic drugs on conditional responses in man*, in: *Neuropsychopharmacology*, E. ROTHLIN (Ed.), Elsevier, Amsterdam.

ALEXANDER, L. (1961 b), Objective evaluation of antidepressant therapy by conditional reflex technique, *Dis. nerv. Syst.*, 22 (5) (Sect. 2, Suppl.), p. 14.

ANANEV, M. G., GOLUMBEVA, L. V., GUROVA, E. V., KASCHEVSKAIA, L. A., LEVITSKAIA, L. A. AND KHUDYI, Y. B. (1960), Preliminary data on experimental electronarcosis induced with apparatus of the scientific research institute of experimental surgical apparatus and instruments, *Anesthesiology*, 21, 215.

ARIETI, S. (Ed.) (1959), *American Handbook of psychiatry*, Basic Books, New York.

ARNOLD, O. H. (1960), Kombinierte Elektroschock – Tofranil Behandlung der Melancholien, *Wien. med. Wschr.*, 110, 250.

ARNOLD, O. H. AND HOFF, H. (1961), Intensive therapy of the psychoneuroses in a university hospital, *Curr. psychiat. Therapy*, 1, 175.

ASHBY, W. Ross (1952), Adrenal cortical function and response to convulsive therapy in a case of periodic catatonia, *J. ment. Sci.*, 98, 81.

BAKER, A. A., BIRD, G., LAVIN, N. I. AND THORPE, J. G. (1960), E.C.T. in schizophrenia, *J. ment. Sci.*, 160, 1506.

BAKER, A. A., GAME, J. A. AND THORPE, J. G. (1958), Physical treatments for schizophrenia, *J. ment. Sci.*, 104, 860.

BARKER, J. C. AND BAKER, A. A. (1959), Deaths associated with electroplexy, *J. ment. Sci.*, 105, 339.

BARRON, D. H. AND MATTHEWS, B. H. C. (1938), The interpretation of potential changes in the spinal cord, *J. Physiol. (Lond.)*, 92, 276.

BEEK, M. VAN DER (1953), *Over de electronarcose-therapie*, Excelsior, 's-Gravenhage.

BENNETT, A. E. (1940), Preventing traumatic complications in convulsive shock therapy by curare, *J. Amer. med. Ass.*, 114, 322.

BLACKER, C. P. (1946), *Neurosis and the mental health services*, Oxford University Press, London.

BLAIR, D. AND BRADY, D. M. (1958), Recent advances in the treatment of schizophrenia: group training and the tranquillizers, *J. ment. Sci.*, 104, 625.

BOCKOVEN, J. S., GREENBLATT, M. AND SOLOMON, H. C. (1951), Treatment results in the major psychoses, *New Engl. J. Med.*, 244, 357.

BOURNE, H. (1953), The insulin myth, *Lancet*, 2, 964.

BOWEN, A. AND CRANE, C. B. (1958), York mental health service, *Frost Report*, 1953-7.

BROWN, G. W., PARKES, C. M. AND WING, J. K. (1961), Admissions and re-admissions to three London mental hospitals, *J. ment. Sci.*, 107, 1070.

CAMBRIDGE UNIVERSITY SYMPOSIUM ON DEPRESSION (1959), Preliminary Report, Cambridge University Press.

CAROTHERS, J. C. (1947), A study of mental derangement in Africans, and an attempt to explain its peculiarities, more especially in relation to the African attitude to life, *J. ment. Sci.*, 93, 548.

CARSE, J. (1959), *The Worthing experiment*, January 1957 to December 1958, a report to the south-west metropolitan regional hospital board.

CERLETTI, U. (1950), L'électrochoc, *Congrès International de Psychiatrie, Paris, Rapports*, Vol. 4, p. 1.

CERLETTI, U. AND BINI, L. (1938), L'électrochoc, *Arch. gen. Neurol. Psychiat.*, 19, 266.

CLEMENT, A. J. (1962), Atropine premedication for electric convulsion therapy, *Brit. med. J.*, 1, 228.

COOK, L. C. (1958), The place of physical treatments in psychiatry, *J. ment. Sci.*, 104, 933.

CRONHOLM, B. AND OTTOSSON, J. O. (1960), Experimental studies of the therapeutic action of electroconvulsive therapy in endogenous depression. The role of the electrical stimulation and of the seizure studied by variation of stimulus intensity and modification by lidocaine of seizure discharge, *Acta psychiat. scand.*, Suppl. 145, p. 69.

CURRAN, D. (1961), The results of psychiatric treatment, *Trans. med. Soc. Lond.*, 78, 72.

DALLY, P. J. AND SARGANT, W. (1960), A new treatment of anorexia nervosa, *Brit. med. J.*, 1, 1770.

DANZIGER, L. AND KINDWALL, J. A. (1946), Prediction of the immediate outcome of shock therapy in dementia praecox, *Dis. nerv. Syst.*, 7, 299.

DAVIES, G. AND PATERSON, A. S. (1952), The use of "etamon" for high blood pressure in electrocerebral treatment, *J. ment. Sci.*, 98, 306.

DELAY, J. (1946), *L'électro-choc et la psychophysiologie*, Masson, Paris.

DELAY, J. (1956), Colloque international sur la chlorpromazine et les médicaments neuroleptiques en thérapeutique psychiatrique: introduction, *Encéphale*, 45, 303.

EDRIDGE, A. (1952), Discussion on new muscle relaxants in electric convulsion therapy, *Proc. roy. Soc. Med.*, 45, 869.

ELLIS, C. H. AND WIERSMA, C. A. G. (1945), Influence of electronarcosis on secretory activity of the pituitary gland, *Proc. Soc. exp. Biol. (N.Y.)*, 58, 160.

FERNANDES, B. AND POLONIO, P. (1946), Indications for the treatment of mental diseases by physical methods, *J. ment. Sci.*, 92, 794.

FREYHAN, F. A. (1961), The influence of specific and non-specific factors on the clinical effects of psychotropic drugs, in: *Neuro-Psychopharmacology*, E. ROTHLIN (Ed.), Elsevier, Amsterdam, Vol. 2, p. 189.

FROSTIG, J. P., HARREVELD, A. VAN, REZNICK, S., TYLER, D. B. AND WIERSMA, C. A. G. (1944), Electronarcosis in animals and in man, *Arch. Neurol. Psychiat. (Chic.)*, 51, 232.

GANTT, W. H. (1950), Disturbances in sexual functions during periods of stress, *Res. Publ. Ass. nerv. ment. Dis.*, 29, 1030.

GARMANY, G. (1958), Depressive states: their aetiology and treatment, *Brit. med. J.*, 2, 341.

GARMANY, G. AND EARLY, D. F. (1948), Electronarcosis, *Lancet*, 1, 444.

GELLHORN, E. (1946), Is restoration of inhibited conditioned reactions by insulin coma specific for pavlovian inhibitions? *Arch. Neurol. Psychiat. (Chic.)*, 56, 216.

GEOGHEGAN, J. J. AND STEVENSON, G. H. (1949), Prophylactic electroshock, *Amer. J. Psychiat.*, 105, 494.

GJESSING, R. (1938), Disturbances of somatic functions in catatonia with a periodic course, and their compensation, *J. ment. Sci.*, 84, 608.

GLOBUS, G. H., HARREVELD, A. VAN, AND WIERSMA, C. A. G. (1943), The influence of electric current application on the structure of the brain of dogs, *J. Neuropath. exp. Neurol.*, 2, 263.

GROSS, M., HITCHMAN, I. C., REEVES, W. P., LAWRENCE, J. AND NEWELL, P. C. (1961), *Discontinuation of treatment with ataractic drugs*, in: *Recent Advances in Biological Psychiatry*, J. WORTIS (Ed.), Grune and Stratton, New York, pp. 44-63.

GUALTIEROTTI, T. (1952), The potential level of the spinal roots during central inhibition and excitation, *J. Physiol., (Lond.)*, 118, 361.

GUALTIEROTTI, T. AND PATERSON, A. S. (1954), Electrical stimulation of the unexposed cerebral cortex, *J. Physiol. (Lond.)*, 125, 278.

GUALTIEROTTI, T. AND PATERSON, A. S. (1956), The physiological effects of non-convulsive bitemporal stimulation in the baboon and man, *Confin. neurol. (Basel)*, 16, 38.

GWATHMEY, J. T. (1914), *Anesthesia*, Appleton, New York.

HALTON, J. (1947), Discussion on further experiences with curare, *Proc. roy. Soc. Med.*, 40, 601.

HARDY, J. D., FABIAN, L. W. AND TWINER, M. D. (1961), Electrical anaesthesia for major surgery: Report of two cases, *J. Amer. med. Ass.*, 175, 599.

HARGREAVES, M. A. (1962), Intravenous atropine premedication before electroconvulsion therapy, *Lancet*, 1, 243.

HARREVELD, A. VAN, AND KOK, D. J. (1934), Über Elektronarkose mittels sinusoidalen Wechselstromes, *Arch. néerl. Physiol.*, 19, 24.

HARREVELD, A. VAN, PLESSET, M. S. AND WIERSMA, C. A. G. (1942), The relation between the physical properties of electric currents and their electronarcotic action, *Amer. J. Physiol.*, 137, 39.

HARRIS, C. R. (1950), Electronarcosis: a safe technique for routine administration under anaesthesia and eulissen (decamethonium iodide or c. 10), *J. ment. Sci.*, 96, 788.

HARTELIUS, H. (1952), Cerebral changes following electrically induced convulsions, *Acta psychiat. scand.*, Suppl. 77.

HASTINGS, D. W. (1961), Circular manic-depressive reaction modified by "prophylactic electroshock", *Amer. J. Psychiat.*, 118, 258.

HAVENS, L. L., ZILLI, M. S., DIMASCIO, A., BOLING, L. AND GOLDFIEN, A. (1959), Changes in catechol amine response to successive electric convulsive treatments, *J. ment. Sci.*, 105, 821.

HILL, D. (1962), Electroencephalography, in: *Recent Advances in Neurology and Neuropsychiatry*, LORD BRAIN (Ed.), 7th ed., J. and A. Churchill, London.

HOBSON, J. A. AND PRESCOTT, F. (1949), Comparison of decamethonium iodide with d-tubocurarine in controlling electrically induced convulsions, *Lancet*, 1, 819.

HOCH, P. H. (1943), Clinical and biological interrelations between schizophrenia and epilepsy, *Amer. J. Psychiat.*, 99, 507.

HOLT, W. L., JR. (1959), Electric vs. chemical tranquillizers in a general hospital private psychiatric practice, *Dis. nerv. Syst.*, 20, 74.

HORDERN, A. (1958), British psychiatry today, *Psychiat. Quart.*, 32, 342.

HORSLEY, J. S. (1936), Narco-analysis, *J. Ment. Sci.*, 32, 416.

IMPASTATO, D. J. (1956), The safer administration of succinylcholine without barbiturates – a new technic, *Amer. J. Psychiat.*, 113, 461.

IMPASTATO, D. J. (1957), Prevention of fatalities in electroshock therapy, *Dis. nerv. Syst.*, 18 (Monograph Suppl.) p. 34.

IMPASTATO, D. (1961), Electric and chemical convulsive therapy in psychiatry (SCC modified EST, metrazol and indoklon convulsive therapy), *Dis. nerv. Syst.*, 22, 91.

JACOBS, G. (1943), Aetiological factors and reaction types in psychoses following childbirth, *J. ment. Sci.*, 89, 242.

JUS, A. (1961), Effect of psychotropic drugs on the C. R. in men and animals, *Neurol. Neurochir. Psychiat. pol.*, 11, 479.

KALINOWSKY, L. B. (1959), *Convulsive shock treatment*, in: *American Handbook of Psychiatry*, S. ARIETI (Ed.), Basic Books, New York, Vol. 2, p. 1499.

KALINOWSKY, L. B. AND HOCH, P. H. (1961), *Somatic treatments in psychiatry*, 3rd Edit., Grune and Stratton, New York.

KALINOWSKY, L. B. AND WORTHING, H. S. (1943), Results with electric convulsive therapy in 200 cases of schizophrenia, *Psychiat. Quart.*, 17, 144.

KIRTSCHEV, K., RAJNOR, A. AND MICHAILOV, S. (1960), Elektroschlaf bei Versuchstieren, *Dtsch. Gesundh.-Wes.*, 15, 1724.

KNUTSON, R. C. (1954), Experiments in electronarcosis: a preliminary study, *Anesthesiology*, 15, 551.

LANCET ANNOTATION (1961), Electrical anaesthesia again, *Lancet*, 1, 1103.

LAPIPE, M. AND RONDEPIERRE, J. (1942), *Contribution a l'étude physique, physiologique et clinique de l'électro-choc*, Maloine, Paris and Montpellier.

LECLERC, G. (1910), L'anesthésie électrique chez l'homme, *Congr. franç. Chir.*, 23, 665.

LEDUC, S. (1902), Production du sommeil et de l'anesthésie générale par les courants électriques, *C. R. Acad. Sci. (Paris)*, 135, 878.

LEDUC, S., MALHERBE, A. AND ROUXEAU, A. (1902), Production de l'inhibition cérébrale chez l'homme par les courants électriques, *C. R. Soc. Biol. (Paris)*, 54, 1297.

LIBERSON, W. T. (1945), Functional electroencephalography in mental disorders, *Dis. nerv. Syst.*, 5, 357.

LILLY, J. C., HUGHES, J. R., ALVORD, E. C. AND GALKIN, T. W. (1955), Brief noninjurious electric waveform for stimulation of the brain, *Science*, 121, 468.

LLOYD, D. P. C. (1941), A direct central inhibitory action of dromically conducted impulses, *J. Neurophysiol.*, 4, 184.

LOPEZ IBOR, J. J. (1950), Indications respectives des méthodes de choc, *Congrès International de Psychiatrie, Paris, 1950, Rapports*, Vol. 4, p. 85.

MACLAY, W. S. (1953), Death due to treatment, *Proc. roy. Soc. Med.*, 46, 13.

MACMILLAN, D. (1956), An integrated mental health service. Nottingham's experience, *Lancet*, 2, 1094.

McWALTER, H. S., MERCER, R., SUTHERLAND, M. AND WATT, A. (1961), Outcomes of treatment of schizophrenia in a north-east Scottish mental hospital, *Amer. J. Psychiat.*, 118, 529.

MALZBERG, B. (1938), Outcome of insulin treatment of 1,000 patients with dementia praecox, *Psychiat. Quart.*, 12, 528.

MEDLICOTT, R. W. (1947), Electronarcosis treatment of schizophrenia, *N.Z. med. J.*, 46, 280.

MEDUNA, L. J. (1937), *Die Konvulsionstherapie der Schizophrenie*, Marhold, Halle.

MEURICE, E. (1960), La polygraphie fonctionnelle peut-elle apporter des critères différentiels pour les malades mentaux, *C. R. Congr. Psychiat. Neurol. Langue franç.*, 58, 427.

MITCHELL, P. H. (1952), Electric convulsion therapy in treatment of prolonged stupor, *Brit. med. J.*, 2, 535.

MONRO, A. B. (1950), Electro-narcosis in the treatment of schizophrenia, *J. ment. Sci.*, 96, 254.

MONTAGU, J. D. (1953), The modification of convulsive therapy by muscle relaxant drugs, *Acta psychiat. scand.*, Suppl. 87.

MOORE, J. N. P. (1960), The treatment of depressive states, with particular reference to imipramine, *Practitioner*, 184, 652.

MORRISSEY, J. AND SAINSBURY, P. (1959), Observations on the Chichester and district mental health service, *Proc. roy. Soc. Med.*, 52, 1061.

MUNCIE, W. (1959), *The psychotherapies: the psychobiological approach*, in: *American Handbook of Psychiatry*, S. ARIETI (Ed.), Basic Books, New York. Vol. 2, p. 1317.

NOACK, C. H. AND TRAUTNER, E. M. (1951), The lithium treatment of maniacal psychosis, *Med. J. Aust.*, 2, 219.

NORRIS, V. (1959), *Mental illness in London*, Maudsley Monograph, No. 6, Chapman, London.

NORTON, A. (1961), Mental hospital ins and outs. A survey of patients admitted to a mental hospital in the past 30 years, *Brit. med. J.*, 1, 528.

OLES, M. (1960), Klinische Erfahrungen mit dem neuroleptikum Haloperidol (R 1625), *Acta neurol. belg.*, 60, 100.

OLTMAN, J. E. AND FRIEDMAN, S. (1961), Comparison of EST and antidepressant drugs in affective disorders, *Amer. J. Psychiat.*, 118, 355.

PALMER, H. A. (1945), Abreactive techniques – ether, *J. roy. Army med. Cps*, 84, 86.

PATERSON, A. S. (1946), Electrical convulsion therapy. Apparatus and indications for use, *Brit. J. phys. Med.*, 9, 8.

PATERSON, A. S. (1948 a), Electro-shock and electronarcosis in the treatment of mental disorders, *Edinb. med. J.*, 55, 38.

PATERSON, A. S. (1948 b), L'électrochoc et l'électronarcose (électrocoma) dans le traitement des troubles mentaux, *Acta neurol. belg.*, 48, 467.

PATERSON, A. S. (1948 c), The technique and application of electronarcosis, *Proc. roy. Soc. Med.*, 41, 575.

PATERSON, A. S. (1952 a), Experiences with electrical stimulation of limited parts of the brain in the baboon and man, *Confin. neurol. (Basel)*, 12, 311.

PATERSON, A. S. (1952 b), E.C.T. for prolonged stupor, *Brit. med. J.*, 2, 723.

PATERSON, A. S. (1958), The failure of emotional development in adolescence as a factor in the causation of schizophrenia, *Congress Report of the IInd. International Congress for Psychiatry, Zurich, Sept. 1957*, Vol. 3, p. 85.

PATERSON, A. S. (1959), The practice of psychiatry in England under the national health service, 1948-59, *Amer. J. Psychiat.*, 116, 244.

PATERSON, A. S. (1960), Types of machine required in electrocerebral treatment, *Third International Conference on Medical Electronics*, London, 1960.

PATERSON, A. S. AND CONACHY, A. (1952), Subconvulsive electrical stimulation in treatment of chronic neurosis, *Brit. med. J.*, 2, 1170.

PATERSON, A. S. AND MILLIGAN, W. L. (1947), Electronarcosis: a new treatment for schizophrenia, *Lancet*, 2, 198.

PERR, I. N. (1961), Psychiatric hospital functioning without EST. A one year study in a state hospital emphasizing intensive treatment, *Arch. gen. Psychiat.*, 4, 479.

PERRIN, G. M. (1961), Cardiovascular aspects of electric shock therapy, *Acta psychiat. scand.,* Suppl. 152.

PICHOT, P. (1960), Vergleich der verschiedenen Behandlungsmethoden in der Psychiatrie (E-Schock, Insulin-Schock, Behandlung mit verschiedenen Neuroleptika allein), *Wien. med. Wschr.,* 110, 734.

PRONKO, N. H., SITTERLY, R. AND BERG, K. (1960), Twenty years of shock therapy in America, 1937-56: an annotated bibliography, *Genet. Psychol. Monogr.,* 62, 233.

REES, L. (1949), Electronarcosis in the treatment of schizophrenia, *J. ment. Sci.,* 95, 625.

RICHTER, C. P. (1931), A biological approach to manic depressive insanity, *Res. Publ. Ass. nerv. ment. Dis.,* 11, 611.

RICHTER, C. P. AND PATERSON, A. S. (1931), Bulbocapnine catalepsy and the grasp reflex, *J. Pharmacol. exp. Ther.,* 43, 677.

RICHTER, C. P. AND PATERSON, A. S. (1932), On the pharmacology of the grasp reflex, *Brain,* 55, 391.

ROBERTSON, G. M. (1926), The prevention of insanity – a preliminary survey of the problem, *J. ment. Sci.,* 72, 454.

ROBINOVITCH, L. G. (1914), in: *Anaesthesia,* J. T. GWATHMEY (Ed.), Appleton, New York, p. 633.

ROKHLIN, L. (1959), *Soviet medicine in the fight against mental diseases,* Lawrence & Wishart, London.

ROTH, M. (1951), Changes in the EEG under barbiturate anaesthesia produced by electroconvulsive treatment and their significance for the theory of ECT action, *Electroenceph. clin. Neurophysiol.,* 3, 261.

ROTH, M. AND ROSIE, J. M. (1953), The use of electroplexy in mental disease with clouding of consciousness, *J. ment. Sci.,* 99, 103.

ROYAL COMMISSION ON THE LAW RELATING TO MENTAL ILLNESS AND MENTAL DEFICIENCY (1954-57) (1957), H. M. Stationery Office, London.

RÜDIN, E. (1927), Erbbiologisch-psychiatrische Streitfragen. *Z. ges. Neurol. Psychiat.,* 108, 274.

RUSSELL, R. J., PAGE, L. G. M. AND JILLETT, R. L., (1953), Intensified electroconvulsive therapy. Review of five years experience, *Lancet,* 2, 1177.

SAKEL, M. (1936), Zur Methodik der Hypoglykämie-Behandlung von Psychosen, *Wien. klin. Wschr.,* 49, 1278.

SARGANT, W. (1942), Physical treatment of acute war neuroses: some clinical observations, *Brit. med. J.,* 2, 574.

SARGANT, W. AND SHORVON, H. J. (1945), Acute war neurosis. Special reference to Pavlov's experimental observations and the mechanism of abreaction, *Arch. Neurol. Psychiat. (Chic.),* 54, 231.

SARGANT, W. AND SLATER, E. (1950), Discussion on the treatment of obsessional neuroses, *Proc. roy. Soc. Med.,* 43, 1007.

SARGANT, W. AND SLATER, E. (1954), *An introduction to physical methods of treatment in psychiatry,* 3rd Edit., E. & S. Livingstone, Edinburgh.

SCURR, C. F. (1951), A relaxant of very brief action, *Brit. med. J.,* 2, 831.

SEAGER, C. P. (1959), Controlled trial of straight and modified electroplexy, *J. ment. Sci.,* 105, 1022.

SELYE, H. (1957), *The stress of life,* Longmans Green & Co., London.

SHEPHERD, M. (1957), *A study of the major psychoses in an English county,* (Maudsley Monographs, No. 3), Chapman & Hall, London.

SLATER, E. (1950), *Mental disorders: heredity,* Chambers Encyclopaedia, Vol. ix, p. 265, Newnes, London.

STENGEL, E. (1959), *Statement at colloquium on depression,* Cambridge.

THORPE, J. G. AND BAKER, A. A. (1958), The effects of physical treatment on some psychological functions, *J. ment. Sci.,* 104, 865.

VETERANS ADMINISTRATION (1956), *Procedure for electro-convulsive treatment,* 2nd Edit., Veterans Administration Center, Neuropsychiatric Hospital, Los Angeles, Calif.

ZEIFERT, M. (1941), Results obtained from the administration of 12,000 doses of metrazol to mental patients, *Psychiat. Quart.,* 15, 772.

PART II

Drug Treatments

Introduction

Development of psychopharmacology in the 1950's

Drugs which act on the brain and nervous system in a selective manner so as to alter emotions and behaviour have been called psychotropic drugs. In the past drugs of this kind, such as opium, scopolamine and the barbiturates had been widely used but the advent of two new compounds, chlorpromazine and reserpine, about 1952, gave a great impetus to the study of pharmacology in relation to nervous and mental disorders.

The discovery of chlorpromazine resulted from the systematic testing out of derivatives of phenothiazine which was carried out in America and France during the 1940's. Phenothiazine itself had been used as a vermifuge and it was hoped further that some derivative would be effective against protozoal infections, but later it was found by the French that one derivative in particular, promethazine (phenergan) had a marked antihistaminic action. The idea that the drug might be useful against schizophrenia was related to a theory that there might exist an allergic form of encephalitis and that this might be responsible for some cases of acute schizophrenia. If this should prove to be so, improvement might be expected from administration of a powerful anti-histaminic agent. However it was later found that another derivative, chlorpromazine, markedly lowered the blood pressure and temperature, as well as potentiating the action of anaesthetics. For this reason chlorpromazine was used in conjunction with pethidine and phenergan as the famous "cocktail" of Laborit (1952), a Parisian surgeon. He not only employed the drug as an adjuvant to anaesthesia but he noticed that when the drug was given alone, patients showed a marked disinterestedness in their surroundings ("indifférence") while they still remained alert. Laborit appreciated the possible value of the drug for excited psychotic patients. However it was Delay and Deniker and their co-workers at the University Clinic of Ste

TABLE III

ACTION OF DIFFERENT CLASSES OF DRUGS ON FUNCTIONAL UNITS IN THE BRAIN

Class	Examples	Cortex	Hypothalamus	Limbic system	Reticular formation
Phenothiazines	Chlorpromazine	Unaffected	Stimulated	Low dose-unaffected High dose-stimulated	Depressed
Rauwolfia	Serpasil	Unaffected	Stimulated	Stimulated	Slightly depressed (high dosag
Diphenylmethane (methonal)	Benactyzine (suavetil) Azacyclonol (frenquel) Hydroxyzine (atarax)	Slightly depressed	Stimulated	Not affected	Slightly depressed
Substituted propanediols	Meprobamate	Not affected	Not affected	Depressed	Not affect or slightly stimulated
Substituted amides	Barbiturates	Depressed	Not affected	Depressed	Depressed

Anne (Delay *et al.*, 1952) who were the first to show the beneficial effects of chlorpromazine when used alone over a long period on schizophrenics. Their work ensured that the remedy became widely known throughout the psychiatric world (Caldwell, 1958).

It was in 1952 also that Mueller, Schlittler and Bein isolated the active alkaloid which they called reserpine (serpasil) from Rauwolfia serpentina Benthami.

For some centuries in India the root of this plant had been used as a remedy for anxiety and excitement. It was called "the insanity root" by the natives. It was first described by the German botanist Rauwolf and the plant was named after him by the Englishman Plumber in 1703. In 1930 Sen and Bose recommended the drug for "insanity and high blood pressure". The first European account of the use of the drug in psychiatry, where it was compared to chlorpromazine, appeared in 1954 by Weber.

(1) The way in which chlorpromazine and serpasil have differed from

their predecessors is that they act mainly on a different area of the brain (Table III). Whereas the barbiturates mainly affect the cortex, these drugs act chiefly on the tegmental reticular system and its connections, and also on the limbic system (the rhinencephalon). They act on the hypothalamus as well, and on the basal ganglia, the autonomic nervous system, the endocrine system and to a lesser extent on the peripheral nerves. They influence the patient's general emotional tone and his degree of spontaneous activity. Their chief characteristics may be tabulated thus: (a) They have a strong sedative effect; (b) there are marked autonomic side effects; (c) a tendency to produce hyperkinetic, dystonic or Parkinsonian symptoms with larger doses; (d) they are suitable for use over a long period in the treatment of schizophrenia.

Drugs belonging to this class, the phenothiazines and Rauwolfia drugs, have been called "neuroleptic drugs" by the French. They have largely taken the place of insulin coma treatment of schizophrenia when combined with ECT (see Rohde and Sargant, 1961; and Sargant, 1958).

(2) In the last few years a second class of drugs has been developed which are sometimes called tranquillisers to distinguish them from the foregoing. Other writers describe chlorpromazine as a tranquilliser and call this group the relaxants. They have the following characteristics: (a) Their sedative action is much less powerful; (b) the autonomic side-effects are negligible; (c) they never produce Parkinsonism; (d) they act on the cortex and subcortical centres equally. The patient's anxiety is greatly reduced, but the reflexes involved, for instance in driving a motor car, are scarcely slowed down at all. Thus meprobamate differs in this respect from alcohol or phenobarbitone. Other relaxants include benactyzine (suavetil) and librium. The last named is proving to be valuable both alone and in conjunction with anti-depressive drugs.

(3) The anti-depressive drugs. About 1951 two drugs were being used in the treatment of tuberculosis which were reported to have a euphoriant effect. One was isoniazid and the other was iproniazid. The second of these, known later as marsilid, had the greater euphoriant action but it was found in a few cases to cause liver damage. It was thought that these drugs owed their euphoriant action to the fact that they were inhibitors of monoamine oxidase and that the degree of euphoria might bear a relation to the level of serotonin in the blood. This was raised by their action. This theory however has not been substantiated. A number of

other monoamine oxidase inhibitors (MAOI's) appeared on the market which were thought to be safer, while retaining the same degree of euphoriant action. However the relationship of the ability to inhibit oxidase to the capacity to ease depression is not yet quite clear, for the best anti-depressants are not MAOI's and some potent MAOI's have only a weak anti-depressive action.

In 1957 an article describing the treatment of depressions with a drug known as imipramine was published (Kuhn 1957). This was later given the trade-name of tofranil. It has a totally different chemical structure from that of iproniazid but it related to chlorpromazine. It may be remarked here that the piperazine derivatives of phenothiazine have a more euphoriant effect than chlorpromazine which in fact can be slightly depressant in its action. Iproniazid (marsilid) however is not used much nowadays. This is on account of its side-effects especially on the liver and it has even been withdrawn from the market in some countries, so that perhaps phenelzine is the most popular of the MAOI's at the present time. However imipramine is more effective against depression than any of the MAOI's. In the last year amitriptyline has become increasingly used and it is claimed that it is more effective against agitation.

(4) Since the beginning of the 1950's considerable interest has been taken in the so-called psychotogenic drugs such as lysergic acid diethylamide (LSD). Mescalin however, a drug with similar effects, had already been tried out in the 1930's. Latterly other drugs such as psilocybin and sernyl have also been investigated. These drugs can now be given with greater safety because chlorpromazine given intravenously acts as an antidote, so that any dangerous effects of the drug can be abolished at once. Chlorpromazine itself however can be dangerous when given by this route unless it is given in only 2.5 per cent solution and administered very slowly. It was hoped that this development would lead to considerable progress in the understanding of mental disorders. Hitherto the psychiatrist has been able only to describe the symptoms of mental disorder but it was now hoped that by investigating temporary and artificial forms of insanity in a laboratory under test conditions ("model psychoses"), more facts would be discovered. It might for instance be possible to correlate a subjective experience like an auditory hallucination with EEG changes in the brain. Although these model psychoses do not exactly resemble those which occur naturally, nevertheless some useful infor-

mation can be elicited from examining the effects of different drugs on the experimental subject.

LSD has also been used as a so-called psycholytic drug, that is, as an adjuvant to psychotherapy. The patient is able to remember more vividly emotionally significant incidents in his past life, which he is able to recount with considerable emotion to the therapist either individually or in groups (Sandison, 1954).

(5) In what follows we shall mention some of the information for which a therapist should look before administering a psychotropic drug, such as indications, dosage range, effects of the drug on animals, side-effects, toxicity and antidotes. We shall also mention the conditions under which clinical trials are carried out. In addition a description will be given of drugs in the above categories as well as a few others. There is an appendix which gives in tabular form the generic name, some trade names, chemical structure, action, indications and side-effects of the various drugs as well as a general assessment of their value.

As this book is intended to be for the use of clinicians, we shall in the following pages frequently refer to drugs by their trade name rather than by their pharmacologically approved name. The trade name is often shorter and more familiar. In the index and the appendix, both the approved names and the trade names are given.

CHAPTER 1

Information Required before Prescribing Psychotropic Drugs

The prescription of psychotropic drugs entails a serious responsibility, for they can affect not only the emotional, cognitive and conative faculties but in the case of some of them moral judgment as well. Only the serious nature of the illness from which the patient suffers, justifies their employment. Mr. Kenneth Robinson, after a world tour, (1961) stated that nearly everywhere he encountered some uneasiness among psychiatrists regarding use of these drugs. It was feared that they were being given by some medical men too indiscriminately and that the ultimate effect on the physical, mental and moral health of the patients was unpredictable.

There are certain points that must be kept in mind in prescribing these agents and in assessing their results. The observations in this Chapter are intended to lessen the chance of the occurrence of ill-effects.

Chemical structure: One should know to which general class the substance belongs and how it differs chemically from other drugs of the same class. For instance stelazine differs from chlorpromazine in having a piperazine side-chain at position 3, as also do fentazin, fluphenazine and some others, and this side-chain is associated not only with a greater degree of potency than chlorpromazine, but also with a greater tendency to energize the patient.

It might be considered illogical to test the so-called "psychotropic" drugs on animals such as rats on the ground that their brains are not sufficiently developed to act as the substratum of a "mind". However the site of feeling and of simple coordination is in the subcortical centres, and these structures are not very different in the lower mammals from in man. These parts, including the brain stem, enable the organism to experience emotions such as pleasure and displeasure, and to be aware of the environment. However owing to the lack of a differentiated forebrain, there is no possibility of logical thinking such as is possible in man, who has the ability to speak.

The following are some methods of studying the central effects of the psychotropic drugs on the lower mammals.

Spontaneous activity: There are various devices for measuring this function in animals. For instance a rat will run inside a wheel so that the wheel revolves. In this way the distance run in 24 hours can be measured. Again one or two rays of light can be directed across a cage and a record can be made of the number of times the animal breaks the beam.

Conditioned motor and visceral reflexes: A rat is put in a cage, the floor of which consists of metal rods. From time to time a light is presented which lasts for several seconds and in the penultimate second the rat experiences a moderately painful shock to the feet, due to the rods on the floor being electrified. In this experiment the unconditioned stimulus (US) is the shock, and the conditioned stimulus (CS) is the light. In the cage there is a vertical stick and as the animal becomes conditioned, the switching on of the light causes him to climb up the little "pole" to avoid the shock.

The animal, which is now given chlorpromazine, reacts differently from the normal animal or from one which has been given nembutal. In the first case the rat pays no attention to the CS but it does to the US, but with nembutal it fails to respond to either the US or the CS. This reaction however is proportional to the degree of hypertonus of muscles or catalepsy and corresponds to the Parkinsonian effect in man. It does not therefore correspond to any therapeutic effect in man but only to the side-effects.

On the other hand one phenothiazine (thioridazine, melleril) does act more markedly on the symptoms of anxiety shown by the animal. The rat to which the light has been presented and which is waiting for the painful shock shows various signs of fear such as piloerection, sweating and tremors. It also tends to void the rectum and the degree of fear is calculated by the number of faecal pellets passed. Under the influence of melleril the animal does not show the flight reaction so readily as normally but it also does not void the rectum as the other rat does despite chlorpromazine.

References p. 221

This experiment (Weidmann, 1961) shows how one may deduce from the behaviour of a rat that melleril would cause little or no Parkinsonian symptoms but would control the morbid emotions of the psychotic, which in fact does occur.

The anti-depressant drugs include compounds which were tried out on man as agents to combat melancholia, because they were found in animals to be inhibitors of monoamine oxidase. The drugs counteracted the lack of energy and apparent depression caused in animals by reserpine. More recent doubts concerning the association of this enzyme with anti-depressive action does not negative the value of much of the work done in this field.

Experiments on animals have thrown light on the pharmacology of tranquillisers such as meprobamate and of chlordiazepoxide (librium). These are blockers of polysynaptic reflexes. The technique here is to show that the drug greatly diminishes the reflex by which the tibialis anterior muscle contracts in response to stimulation of the central end of the cat's severed tibial nerve. On the other hand the monosynaptic patellar reflex is hardly affected. This type of drug has also an anti-convulsive effect. In high doses it does not cause sleep but rather ataxia in the same manner as alcohol.

Lysergic acid diethylamide (LSD) has a sympathomimetic effect, with piloerection, mydriasis, hyperthermia, tachycardia, tachypnoea and hyperglycaemia. In animals sensitivity to external stimuli is enhanced. Thus when a painful heat stimulus is applied to the tail of a mouse, the reflex of moving the tail is carried out much more quickly when the animal is under the influence of LSD. This over-sensitivity to external stimuli causes a fall in the spontaneous activity of animals if there is a normal amount of light and sound. If however they are cut off from external stimuli their spontaneous activity is not impaired. The lowering of the threshold to both external and visceroceptive stimuli is probably the basis of its hallucinogenic action.

The macac monkey is particularly suitable for studying the degree and duration of cataleptic state, which corresponds to a Parkinsonian condition in man (Richter and Paterson, 1932; de Jong, 1945).

A new science has sprung up which may one day be of great value to the psychiatrist. This is the field of microbiochemistry (McIlwain, 1959). Such abstruse matters as the electrical potential outside a cell membrane in relation to that inside is of importance. Also the passage of sodium in and out of the cell body. The metabolic rate of a cell can be measured, and even the concentration of a substance in the mitrochondria of a cell can be estimated.

The science of electroencephalography has also given information on the site of action of various drugs. By means of it light has been thrown on the mesodiencephalic activating system and on the limbic system in animals. These have been important for the understanding of the action of the phenothiazines.

Indications and target symptoms: Some knowledge of the experiments reported on animals with regard to a particular drug gives an idea of what the target symptoms are in man, which it is hoped will be removed by the drug. The three main classes of psychotropic drugs are those used for schizophrenia, those for depression and those for anxiety neurosis.

The drugs which influence schizophrenia decrease feelings of persecution and ideas of reference. They tend to remove oneiric or dreamlike thinking which is irrational and which follows the laws of free association. The drug may make it possible for the patient to employ rational and logical thinking again. Further, with the abolition of dream-thinking and with the onset of a calmer attitude the delusions and hallucinations may also disappear.

Behavioural adjustment scales: The clinical psychiatrist can obtain more satisfaction from this type of work if he constructs his own questionnaire in which he records all the symptoms observed before treatment is given and compares them with the symptoms during and after treatment. In such a rating scale emphasis is laid on biological as well as subjective symptoms. In large-scale clinical trials carried out by a team, clinical psychologists generally employ recognised rating scales.

In the same way, a questionnaire can be drawn up and multiplicated for investigating patients suffering from cyclothymic disorders. Here again questions relating to appetite, sleep, changes of weight and spontaneous activity, as well as subjective events such as feelings and emotions can be recorded. Often the questionnaire can be handed to the wife of the patient who can record when symptoms change. Relatives can write up the order of the disappearance of the symptoms of melancholia, such as constipation, insomnia, loss of appetite and the onset of increased activity with the loss of depression and suicidal thoughts.

Similarly a questionnaire can be composed for patients who are suffering from states of anxiety and tension including obsessional symptoms. An account of the order of disappearance of the numerous somatic symptoms can be accurately recorded.

Dosage: A note is made of the minimal dose which is said to be effective and the maximal dose which can be given without side-effects or at least serious ones. Some indication of the drug's toxicology can be obtained by seeing the difference between the effective dose in animals and the LD_{50} (*i.e.* the dose which is lethal to 50 per cent of animals of the species tested).

One should know if there is any record in the literature of a suicidal attempt with an over-dose of the drug in question and if a large dose was consistent with survival. Librium for instance can be taken in large doses without causing death, as also the soporific melsedin.

One of the commonest errors is to give the drug in a dose which is lower than the threshold. An American psychiatrist has said that the most prevalent placebo or drug of suggestion used in general practice at the present time is a neuroleptic drug which is given below the threshold of effectiveness (Kline, 1961).

In the case of some drugs a low dose can have a very different effect from a relatively high one. This is illustrated by the phenomenon of turbulence which occurs with the Rauwolfia drugs and with some of the piperazine derivatives.

One should know if idiosyncrasies have been reported. Occasionally an allergic reaction such as angioneurotic oedema can occur with meprobamate. Very occasional cases have been reported of collapse after as little as 25 or 50 mg of chlorpromazine. Less well known is the danger of giving chlorpromazine intravenously even in 2.5 per cent solution. We have seen the collapse of a volunteer after an intravenous injection of chlorpromazine which was given to counteract the effects of psilocybin, but revival occurred after the injection of nikethamide and elevation of the patient's feet. Again, one should know that thioridazine should not be given in doses of over 600 mg a day. Cases have been reported of retinopathy with very high doses.

Side-effects: We have gained information about symptoms not ordinarily reported about certain drugs from questionnaires given to patients. For instance, complaints are made of the smell of the sweat from medication with imipramine. If the patient takes 75 mg at one time the taste may remain with him for as long as 12 hours. The bed in which he has been sleeping has a peculiar smell if the patient has sweated much.

One should know whether a drug leads to tolerance, *i.e.* whether after a while a larger dose becomes necessary. This can happen with chlorpromazine; also if it can lead to habitation or addiction, which can occur with meprobamate.

If it is desired to prolong the action of a drug taken by mouth, this can be often effected by providing the drug in coated granules (called by one firm spansules). Again, if a drug takes rather a long time to act, or if it is destroyed to a certain extent in the stomach, then it can be given intramuscularly. We have a definite impression that imipramine acts more rapidly by the intramuscular route and amitriptyline is often given by this route also.

One should know if the action of a drug continues, as that of MAOI's do for days or even weeks after they have been stopped. This is important because it is dangerous for a patient to have an anaesthetic if he is under the influence of an MAOI drug.

The MAOI drugs and the drugs with powerful Parkinsonian action (fluphenazine, majeptil, haloperidol) should be used with the utmost caution.

Literature: One should know if any controlled trials have been carried out and if they are reliable, and if they indicate that the drug is valuable. If two drugs are about the same in effectiveness, it may be found that one is less dangerous and freer from side-effects and therefore preferable.

Laboratory test: In our clinic we have a conditioned reflex set-up for simultaneous recording of physiological functions by means of five cathode-ray oscilloscopes. This type of investigation has given interesting data in connection with the action of drugs in man as has been shown both by Alexander (1961 a and b) and Paterson *et al.* (1962).

Conclusion: Psychotropic drugs are still thought to be best classified on the basis of their chemical structure. It is therefore advisable that the psychiatrist should know something about the class of drug which is employed. If he is acquainted with the pharmacology and with the target symptoms for which the drug is intended, he will use it more effectively. It is however advisable that he should know the effects of low, medium and high dosage, since the effects may vary with the amount given. Many clinical trials are carried out with two or three different doses. He should also know what toxic effects and side-effects may be caused in susceptible individuals. Finally, he should be acquainted with the general assessment of the drug made by competent authorities on the basis of controlled trials (see Am. Med. Ass., Council on Drugs, 1959; Extra Pharmacopoea, 1958, also supplement, 1961 and Cole *et al.*, 1961).

CHAPTER 2

The Technique of Clinical Trials

The first clinical trial in which matched controls were employed was probably the experiment carried out by James Lind in 1747 who proved that the juices of oranges and lemons could prevent scurvy (Green, 1954). Since this early start the British have developed this technique and made it peculiarly their own. It has suited the national character which is apt to adopt a sceptical attitude towards press reports of the sensational effects of some new drug. By 1931 the Medical Research Council had formed a Therapeutic Trials Committee to try out new drugs, which tests in the laboratory had shown to have a probable therapeutic value. In 1936 they proved the value of prontosil when it was hardly out of its experimental stage in Germany, the country of its origin. In the 1940's Bradford Hill and his colleagues organised trials on penicillin and later on the triad streptomycin, PAS and isoniazid which nowadays save some 60,000 lives a year in Great Britain from tuberculosis.

It was therefore fortunate for psychiatrists that when psychotropic drugs appeared in the 1950's, the science of clinical trials had already reached a stage of development which made an assessment of their value more accurate than would otherwise have been the case. There is however a difference between a trial designed to investigate whether a drug destroys a micro-organism and one which removes the symptoms of disordered behaviour and distressing subjective symptoms. The patient has, as it were, a pre-arranged "set", in virtue of which he reacts to indifferent stimuli by suspicion and rage or by intense fear, or again by uninhibited over-activity and elation, or by inaction and depression with suicidal impulses, or again by the archaic reaction-pattern of catatonia. Patients who suffer from these disorders may show a remarkable remission of symptoms following the administration, for a period, of one or other of the psychotropic drugs. It is however more difficult to assess to what extent the drug is having a direct effect on the nervous system of the patient so

References p. 221

as to cause the recovery, and how far extraneous factors are entering into the process. Three other factors in addition to the specific action of the drug may produce the change (see Witts, 1959).

(1) The placebo effect: The placebo is an inert drug which is given to patients generally as a control, with which the presumably active drug can be compared. Occasionally it is a drug which imitates the side-effects of the active drug. In 1955 Beecher made a series of 15 studies on 1082 patients suffering from physical and psychiatric illness and found the average efficiency of a placebo to be 32.2 per cent, while Kurland (1957) using a smaller but exclusively psychiatric sample showed a range of 4-52 per cent of recoveries. In England Tibbetts and Hawkings (1956) comparing the effects of CO_2 therapy and compressed air, reported an improvement rate of 50 per cent with both methods, while again the effects of intravenous acetylcholine showed a recovery rate of 60 per cent but so also did the patients who were injected with sterile water.

The psychology of the placebo-reactor is not completely understood. According to some writers he is not merely a hysterical individual who is anxious to please his doctor but a conscientious church-going type with an optimistic outlook. He is introvert rather than extrovert and he is presumably suggestible to the extent that he is affected by the image of himself once more restored to health (Trouton, 1957).

(2) Milieu effect: When working in the Middlesex Hospital sector of the Emergency Medical Service in the London area 1939-1943, I had the opportunity of working part-time at St. John's Hospital, Aylesbury, which is a large mental institution. During that period there was intense activity by Dr. Edith Booth and others in applying convulsive therapy to a large number of patients, mostly schizophrenics and cyclothymics. Not only did recent patients respond well but a number of patients who had been in the hospital for many years, especially involutional melancholics, recovered and returned home. These events made some impression on the neighbouring community. They were indeed made possible by the initiative shown by the Medical Superintendant, I. Skottowe who had not only been using insulin coma in the 1930's but had organised a psychiatric service by which patients were seen at an early stage in their illness either as out-patients in the local general hospital or at home. He had also

improved the amenities of the hospital. It was noticed however that not only the patients treated with ECT but some others whose condition had remained stationary, began to show improved behaviour and began to talk about returning to the outside world.

The new enthusiasm, generated by the success of shock treatments, among the medical and nursing staff and the humanitarian approach which followed it, created a milieu which was favourable to the patient's recovery. The patient was trusted with more freedom. He was given a new dignity and felt he was living in a kindly world.

In order to ensure that the milieu effect is not confused with the drug effect, one must have control groups. Those receiving the inert drug and those being given the active drug are both subjected to the same conditions. This point has been emphasised by Rathod (1961).

(3) Inter-action effect: This describes the attitude of the patient to the effect of the drug on the target symptoms. In most cases this would be expected to be favourable and the patient is likely to report that he is feeling much better. Often however a better criterion of improvement is the report of the patient's family or of the nursing staff in his ward.

Some patients have lost heart and adopt a deep-seated attitude which indicates "I am not going to play". These are the hypochondriacs who run the gamut of all the treatments including leucotomy and may even end by committing suicide. One such man who bungled his only chance of promotion in life, talked repeatedly of suicide for years afterwards and refused to work. At first he had the classical symptoms of depression, insomnia, anorexia, failure of concentration, etc. but these remitted with ECT. Later when given anti-depressive drugs he insisted that like ECT they had no effect on him and yet his wife reported that at a bridge tournament the night before he had been the life and soul of the party. Another patient with involutional melancholia reported that she was steadily improving up to the 7th ECT, but after the 8th an apparent relapse occurred. It was found that she had taken a sudden dislike to the psychiatrist. She returned a week later to say that she had been miraculously cured by a faith-healer.

(4) Specific effect of the drug: Constitutional and physical factors play a greater role in the psychoses, where abnormal behaviour is less easily

reversed by psychotherapy, than in the neuroses. The psychiatrist thinks of the patient more in biological terms. If the patient is depressed, we ask about spontaneous activity, the number of hours of sleep, and whether the patient takes long to fall asleep or wakens early, the amount of food he eats, and the amount of weight he has lost. Measurements are introduced wherever possible. Patients are sometimes even asked to carry pedometers to record the distance walked in the day.

In schizophrenia a record is made of the degree of catalepsy, the amount of aggressive or destructive behaviour, or inaction, as well as of sleep and appetite. We record also the degree to which the patient can take part in communal activity and how far his thinking is of an archaic or autistic type and how far it is at the rational and logical level.

It is sometimes said that the effect of the phenothiazines on schizophrenia is not specific but they do have a tranquillizing effect, and in the case of the piperazines a euphoriant action as well. Delusions and hallucinations disappear just as they do when chlorpromazine is given to a subject who has hallucinations caused by LSD.

In consequence of these effects the patient looks and feels more normal and the clinician can establish rapport with him. In time the patient acquires a more satisfactory relationship to his fellows and to his work.

Even if this is said not to be a specific effect on the disease process, the phenothiazines at least cause a remission of the characteristic symptoms of schizophrenia in a manner which has not been equalled by any other class of drug up to the present time.

The uncontrolled trial   This often takes the form of a preliminary or pilot experiment, the aim of which is to obtain a general impression of the action of a drug prior to the carrying out of a more elaborate and costly controlled trial. The value of this is greater when it is applied to chronic patients who have not reacted to previous methods of treatment. If there is an apparent marked improvement which follows closely on the heels of the new drug, there is a strong presumption that the drug is in fact active.

Although some psychiatrists prefer to draw up their own rating scale, especially adjusted for the particular study, there are a number of scales which have been published, including the MACC behavioural adjustment scale described by Ellsworth and Clayton (1959).

Some drugs which are already established are so successful in removing distressing symptoms, that unless a new drug appears to have a much more definite effect on the target symptoms, it is not likely that the trouble and expense of a time-consuming controlled trial would be considered justifiable.

The controlled trial Where this is proposed, a considerable amount of time should be devoted to working out the details of the project. This often has a main object and two or three subsidiary objects. At one stage it would be necessary to discuss with a statistician the most convenient way of studying the clinical material. Care taken at this stage will save an immense amount of labour later on. If the project is well designed, even although it is elaborate in some respects, there would be a maximum economy of effort in the long run, with valid conclusions from the data investigated. Some workers can almost write an account of the whole experiment before it is undertaken, leaving only the figures to be filled in. Generally however unforeseen complications interfere with the smooth running of the project. Duties are assigned to different members of the team and an attempt is made to adhere strictly to a time schedule.

Marley (1959) has analysed 15 recent trials reported in British journals with regard to the drug tested, the range of dosage, the diagnosis, target symptoms, sex, method of control, the fact whether doctors, patients or nurses made the assessment, statistics and results.

The following are some points which should be noted. The investigator should indicate clearly what the target symptoms are and what effect the drug had on them. The sex of the patient should always be mentioned. There is a common view that the phenothiazines for instance act more favourably on women.

Types of trial In a number of trials two groups of patients are used who are matched as far as possible for age, diagnosis and duration of their illness. The allotment of the patient to the treated group or to the controlled group should be random. Sometimes the spin of a coin is used. The bigger that the two groups are, duration of illness etc. will cancel each other out as between the two groups.

Sometimes the patients are used as their own controls. After a definite period the control group can then be given the drug while the treated group then receives the placebo. In more complicated trials other groups can be added, one of which receives a different drug, the efficacy of which has already been well established. Rees and Lambert (1955) who used the cross-over technique write "The method of using the patient as his own control has much to recommend it, especially if such methods as the double blind and sequence control procedures are utilised, enabling the effect of suggestion to be ascertained, and also the control of factors unrelated to the pharmacological effects of the drug."

In the double blind technique neither the doctors nor nursing staff know whether the placebo or the active drug is being given in a particular case. The numbers of the staff however generally know when the switch-over takes place. It is generally the hospital pharmacist who keeps a record of the medication assigned to each patient. The virtue of the double blind technique as indicated already is that it prevents the placebo effect from occurring in the patients and prevents any bias on the part of the staff in recording results. The disadvantage of the cross-over method is that some drugs may have a cumulative effect which persists into the placebo period. These objections have more relevance when there is a switch-over from the first drug to a second drug. This last drug's action may be modified by a hang-over from the effect of the first drug, or the first drug may have effected a recovery which is attributed to the second drug.

Usually a short period intervenes between the two drugs or again a placebo period can intervene.

Dosage   Ideally there should be at least two dose levels and each of these should be alternated with the placebo. This increases the likelihood that one of the doses will fall in the steepest part of the dose-response curve for the group. The results would be more accurate if the dosages were calculated per unit of body weight. Some trials are sufficiently elaborate for 3 dose-levels to be employed, so that a dose-response regression and the relative potencies of the different drugs can be calculated. If two or more dose-levels are used, then they should be related geometrically to each other, as geometric increments or decrements of dose are associated with arithmetic increase or decrease of drug response (Marley, 1959).

Analysis of results   An expert will be able to help in choosing the statistical criteria indicated in a particular trial where quantitative data are available. Analysis with X^2 means a loss of potential information, as this is a test strictly for a homogeneous experimental population. In comparing two groups of mentally ill patients, a number of different factors contributes to variability in the response to drugs and the use of the "t" test which only distinguishes between inter-group differences precludes any elucidation except the summed effect of these variables. A more complicated procedure is described by Fisher (1950). It is called the Analysis of Variance and is an extension of the "t" test. It is often used where more than two variables are to be compared.

A fact not widely known is that valid results can be obtained in certain types of trial with relatively small groups of patients, such as thirty, if the correct statistical methods are employed. See Armitage (1950).

Drawbacks and fallacies of controlled trials

Unless a controlled trial is well designed and efficiently carried out, the immense amount of time consumed and the monetary expense involved will to a great extent have been wasted. Many errors can occur. Allusion has already been made to some of these, such as wrong dosage, application of unsuitable statistical technique, a careless selection of patients from the diagnostic standpoint, a too rapid cross-over from the use of one drug to another and so on.

Another fallacy has been caused by temporary side-effects. When Rauwolfia is given, there is often a preliminary period of "turbulence" when the patient appears to be much worse and this in some cases has led to adverse reports on its final action. Perhaps not enough attention has been paid to the influence of transitory side-effects on the judgment of medical observers in judging the ultimate effect of the drug. Freyhan (1961 a), for instance, in assessing the relative efficacy of a number of phenothiazine derivatives (he includes reserpine as well) rates thioridazine highest and majeptil and reserpine about lowest. His "therapeutic ratio" is the relation of the number of patients showing optimal changes to those showing failure. Fluphenazine which also shows marked side-effects has the poorest results after promazine in this series, followed in turn by trifluoperazine (stelazine). It is possible that if anti-Parkinsonian drugs had been administered or if the dose in each case had been carefully

References p. 221

adjusted, so as to be just below the level where Parkinsonian or other disagreeable extra-pyramidal symptoms appear, the rating would have been different.

Conclusion

A great deal of satisfaction can be obtained by the clinician even if he is not working in a university clinic or research centre by reading the whole literature relating to the drugs which he is using. He will find interest in compiling suitable questionnaires to be filled up before, during and after treatment is given. He can apply one of the many rating scales which record continuous improvement or otherwise. The construction of these has reached a greater degree of elaboration in the USA than elsewhere and an attempt is made to make them as reliable as possible. No large-scale clinical trial is carried out without the use of such scales. Lorr (1960) has given a good account of these. It is also an interesting experience for the younger psychiatrist when he takes part in a team effort in which a successful project is carried through to the end and a useful contribution has been added to the sum of psychiatric knowledge.

CHAPTER 3

Rauwolfia Alkaloids

Reserpine (serpasil)

The alkaloid which is most commonly used is reserpine (serpasil). Its chemical structure is given in the appendix. It has affinities both with serotonin and also with some of the psychotogenic drugs such as mescalin, psilocybin and LSD. It is known that reserpine lowers the serotonin content of the brain within a short period by 90 per cent. It has also been found that the level of noradrenaline in the brain is reduced. The question whether the neuroleptic effects of reserpine are related to its ability to lower the content of serotonin and noradrenaline in the brain has not yet been decided.

The finding that reserpine does not begin to act for some hours or days and that its action continues after withdrawal of the drug leads one to suppose that the effect is not direct upon the brain but indirect through its action on some naturally occurring substance. It is thought that this substance is in fact serotonin. Brodie *et al.* (1960) wrote as follows: "Reserpine impairs the mechanism that maintains serotonin in a stored form, but does not affect its rate of synthesis. Thus the free amine continues to be made, but now can freely diffuse from sites of synthesis. Serotonin is rapidly synthesised in the brain, so despite its breakdown by monoamine oxidase, the level at synapses may be higher after reserpine administration than before. Reserpine action in the brain may result therefore from a continuous release of serotonin on the receptor sites."

Effects on animals

It has a central effect and to a lesser degree it acts on the periphery as well. It inhibits the sympathetic so that there is parasympathetic predominance, as shown by meiosis, bradycardia, low blood pressure, increased peristalsis and diarrhoe. It can have an emetic effect.

Extrapyramidal symptoms consist of restlessness, which is transitory, and catatonia in animals. In man the catatonia is replaced by Parkinsonism.

It has a sedative effect on animals and reduces their spontaneous activity. The depression caused by the drug is used to test the energizing effect of the so-called monoamine oxidase inhibitors.

Dosage

The drug has been given intramuscularly or intravenously as well as orally. It has been given intravenously, 5 mg in 2 ml, but at least one death has been reported. By this route it does not act before the lapse of an hour, so it is useless in an acute emergency. If the drug is given i.m. (5 mg) the effect will not be obtained any quicker than by the oral route.

The psychotic patient is generally given 3 mg by mouth daily for 10 days. Some workers give 5 to 10 mg i.m. at night to start the patient off. High doses appear to be dangerous on account of the possibility of an ulcer. Parkinsonism is generally caused by doses of over 5 mg. For outpatients the dosage recommended is generally 0.25 mg t.d.s. up to 1 mg t.d.s. but for hospitalised patients much higher doses have been given. For very disturbed patients as much as 5 mg t.d.s. has been given but cardiac complications as well as a perforated gut can result.

Indications

Reserpine is especially indicated for chronic schizophrenics in a mental hospital on account of its sedative effect, which is not as a rule accompanied by somnolence or ataxia. The patient remains alert and interested in his environment. However it does not abolish hallucinations and delusions as effectively as chlorpromazine. It is also useful in excitement of its sedative effect.

Main differences from chlorpromazine

(1) Chlorpromazine acts rapidly whereas reserpine is slow in its action.

(2) After chlorpromazine has been used for about 1 or 2 weeks, habituation tends to occur but this does not occur with reserpine. (3) Chlorpromazine has little or no effect on the patient's mood, whereas reserpine may cause depression. (4) Chlorpromazine does not cause the same degree of Parkinsonism or "turbulence" as does reserpine. (5) The side-effects are different. With an overdose of chlorpromazine there is a tendency for the patient to collapse. There may be some oedema and there may be jaundice and allergic reactions. With reserpine however the dangers are of low blood pressure, the formation of peptic ulcers, and colic from excessive peristalsis. (6) Chlorpromazine acts more on the tegmental reticular substance whereas reserpine acts more on the limbic system.

Reserpine is used in some mental hospitals for mania because of its depressant and sedative effect.

The effects of the drug continue for quite a long time after it has been withheld and this should be remembered when other drugs are prescribed, as when the patient has to receive an anaesthetic.

After the drug has ceased to take effect, the symptoms may return and only about one-fifth of the patients who have been treated for schizophrenia remain well after it has been withdrawn and the effects of the drug have worn off.

Barsa and Kline (1955) have described three stages in the course of treatment with serpasil. The first is a sedative stage in which the patient is quiet and drowsy and this lasts from 3 to 10 days. His appetite improves and he may gain weight. There is then a turbulent stage in which the patient becomes more disturbed and there is an exacerbation of delusions and hallucinations. This stage has caused some confusion for research workers who have received reports from nursing attendants that patients are made worse by the drug. However if this treatment is persisted in for another three weeks, then the third stage is reached which is called the integrative stage in which the patient becomes more co-operative, friendly and interested in his surroundings.

If a patient is being given insulin coma treatment and it is difficult to get the patient into a state of coma, a little reserpine will help to achieve this result.

References p. 221

Other alkaloids and congeners

Most reports state that reserpine is the most effective alkaloid of the
Rauwolfia group but Malamud *et al.* (1957) found that although reserpine
gave the best results at the end of treatment, after 6 months rescinnamine
gave better results.

Deserpidine has a more rapid action but is generally thought to be less
potent. Lethargy and mental depression are less marked. The doses are the
same as with reserpine.

Raudixin is a preparation of the whole root and the dose is therefore
much higher, being 100 mg *t.d.s.*

Tetrabenazine (nitoman) is a synthetic drug. It has central effects
resembling those of reserpine. Unlike reserpine it appears to have very
little peripheral activity and its effects persist for only 24 to 36 hours. It
has been said to cause the disappearance of hallucinations and delusions.
It has a marked sedative action. It is well tolerated and the principal side-
effects are transient restlessness and drowsiness. With a high dose Parkinsonism can occur. It should not be used with reserpine or immediately
after a course of a MAOI drug. The initial daily dose is 100 to 150 mg but
this can be increased if necessary up to 200 mg. The daily maintenance
dose is 50 to 75 mg. Kanjilal and Matheson (1962) have reported favourably on the use of this drug in low grade mental defectives.

CHAPTER 4

Phenothiazines

We have already described the place of the phenothiazines in the general class of psychotropic drugs. Chlorpromazine, the original member of this group may be taken as the yardstick by which to measure the effectiveness of its successors. During recent years a large number of phenothiazine derivatives have appeared on the market, partly because on rare occasions serious side-effects such as agranulocytosis or hepatic damage have been reported with chlorpromazine (Meyler, 1960), and partly because similar drugs have been found to be more effective. In some instances the structural modifications of chlorpromazine have resulted in a reduction in the incidence of dangerous side-effects but at the price of diminished clinical effectiveness, while an increased potency and energising effect have been accompanied by a disagreeable increase in extrapyramidal symptoms. For instance, the removal of the chlorine radical at position 2 in the central ring of chlorpromazine and addition of hydrogen gives promazine (sparine) and reduces its toxicity but diminishes its therapeutic effectiveness (Rathod, 1961). A more successful change was the substitution of a trifluoromethyl group for the chlorine radical. This reduced the danger of side-effects while maintaining the clinical efficiency (vespral).

Other changes in the chlorpromazine molecule have been effected through modification of the dimethyl-aminopropyl side chain*. For the most part these alterations have resulted not only in giving the compound an increased potency but also an increased propensity to produce extrapyramidal symptoms. For instance the substitution of a piperazine side-chain for a dimethylaminopropyl chain (prochlorperazine, stemetil) gives a compound which is 5 to 10 times more potent than chlorpromazine but increases some extra-pyramidal symptoms such as acathisia. These piperazines are perphenazine (fentazin), prochlorperazine (stemetil), thiopro-

---

* Compare text with appendix throughout the following Chapters.

pazate (dartalan) and trifluoperazine (stelazine). These all have similar effects.

The two drugs which are most potent in producing Parkinsonian symptoms are fluphenazine (moditen) which is a piperazine, and also thioproperazine (majeptil), are both piperazinyl derivatives.

The justification of these last two drugs is that they are possibly more effective in severe cases of schizophrenia, where other drugs of this class have failed. We shall discuss the problem of how best to produce the maximal therapeutic effect with a phenothiazine drug while at the same time diminishing the unpleasant extrapyramidal side-effects to a minimum.

A further development in the last few years has been the discovery of two drugs which are potent therapeutically in some cases of schizophrenia but which produce minimal Parkinsonian side-effects. These are thioridazine (melleril) and chlorprothixene (taractan, truxal). Melleril has the phenothiazine ring but a piperidine side-chain at position 10 while chlorprothixene has a thioxanthene ring structure. Instead of the trivalent nitrogen atom in the central ring there is a carbon atom which is attached by two bonds to the same side-chain as in chlorpromazine. This drug also has much the same anti-depressive action as imipramine.

It is thought that the sedative effect of this class of drug depends on the three carbon atoms in the side-chain being in line between the central ring and the terminal radical. Promethazine (phenergan) does not have the same sedative effect and has only two carbon atoms in line.

The typical effect of chlorpromazine is to reduce excitement, agitation, feelings of persecution and delusions as well as hallucinations. At the same time it does not typically produce a drowsy or sleepy state. On the other hand it is not indicated for neurotic anxiety which it may even intensify. A curious property of the piperazines such as stelazine and fentazin is that they have an energizing effect as well as a sedative one.

The best policy for a clinician is to concentrate mostly on one drug and to employ others only in cases where this one is not suitable. In our clinic we have used fentazin as the representative of this group more than any other.

Pharmacology of the phenothiazines

Two diagrams, figs. 8 and 9, show the sites in the brain where the phenothiazines act. It is possible to divide the whole brain into structurally different regions which have separate functions. There are four main regions. These are the cortex, the hypothalamus, the limbic system and the reticular formation. Cortical activity is necessary for the functions of thought and judgment. The effects of a drug on the function of the cortex

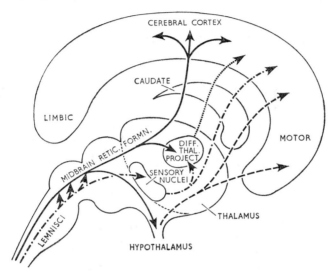

Fig. 8. Mesodiencephalic activating system. Stimulation of the organism evokes impulses which travel by way of the lemnisci to the thalamic sensory nuclei and thence to cortical sensory areas. The lemnisci send collateral nerve fibres to the mid-brain reticular formation and by these fibres, impulses pass in the reticular formation to the diffuse thalamic projections and excite the cerebral cortex. Collaterals bearing stimuli from the midbrain reticular formation pass to the hypothalamus, which in turn sends impulses to the cerebral cortex (after Himwich, 1960, reprinted with permission).

can sometimes be deduced if one observes its effects on the EEG. The group of drugs which acts chiefly on the cortex is that of the barbiturates. The EEG shows a decrease in the frequency of the rhythm and an increase in the voltage, giving a pattern similar to that observed during natural sleep.

The hypothalamus is the centre from which all autonomic functions are controlled. The phenothiazines as well as the Rauwolfia alkaloids and the diphenylmethanes, which include suavitil (benactyzine), aza-cyclonal (frenquel) and hydroxyzine (atarax) have a stimulant effect on these hypothalamic centres. This is shown by their ability to lower the convulsive threshold to ECT, and to increase the effects of strychnine, which is known to heighten the excitability of the posterior sympathetic nuclei of the hypothalamus.

The action of the phenothiazines in schizophrenia is thought to be

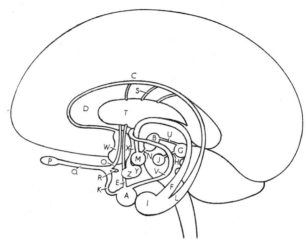

Fig. 9. Semidiagrammatic section of human brain. A. amygdala; B. anterior nucleus of thalamus; C. cingulate gyrus; D. corpus callosum; E. diagonal band (Broca); F. Fornix; G. habenula; H. habenulopeduncular tract; I. hippocampus; J. interpeduncular nucleus; K. lateral olfactory stria; L. longitudinal stria; M. mammillary body; N. mammillothalamic tract; O. medial olfactory stria; P. olfactory bulb; Q. olfactory tract; R. olfactory tubercle; S. perforating fibres; T. septum pellucidum; U. stria medullaris; V. stria terminalis; W. subcallosal gyrus; X. hypothalamus; Y. posterior pituitary gland; Z. anterior pituitary gland.

partly due to this action, for the functions of the hypothalamus are much inhibited in this disorder.

The limbic system (Fig. 9) which is also known as the rhinencephalon or visceral brain is situated rostrally to the hypothalamus and it is of vital importance for processes related to emotion. Anatomically it consists of the hippocampus, the amygdala, the fornix, the olfactory cortex and related structures. The action of drugs in this region of the brain is studied by analysing spontaneous potentials and by observing the occurrence and duration of after-discharges which have been produced by local electrical stimulation (Preston, 1956). Phenothiazines (Killam and Killam, 1957) also produce seizure discharges in this system. These high amplitude discharges remain confined to the limbic system and do not spread readily to other areas. If however the dose is greatly increased, the seizures may spread to the cortex in which case the animal has a convulsion (Kinross-Wright, 1955). If a drug is applied locally to the limbic system in such a way that localised seizures occur, then the behaviour of the animal is the same as if it is receiving chlorpromazine or reserpine. It is surprising that the seizures are related to a sedating effect. There is in fact a poverty of spontaneous movements. The animal does not respond to a conditioned stimulus.

The propanediols (such as meprobamate) and the hypnotics like the barbiturates do not alter the spontaneous potentials in the limbic structure, but they abolish or shorten after-discharges which have been set up by electrical stimulation in this area.

The reticular formation which is partly in the brain stem and partly in the tegmentum controls wakefulness and sleep. A pain stimulus will affect this area and so arouse a resting animal and produce a so-called arousal reaction in the EEG as picked up from the cortex. The propanediols such as meprobamate do not block the reaction in the reticular formation but may even slightly stimulate it. The phenothiazines have the effect of depressing this structure and inhibiting the arousal reaction but the effect of the Rauwolfia drugs is negligible in ordinary doses (Himwich, 1960).

Chlorpromazine has some anti-adrenergic effects such as lowering the blood pressure, though it does not inhibit the hyperglycaemic response to adrenalin. It potentiates the action of barbiturates and of morphia and counteracts the effects of caffeine and amphetamine but not of strychnine. There is a reduction in the spontaneous activity of the subject (Taeschler and Schlager, 1961).

Technique of treatment with phenothiazines

Treatment with largactil has been described in Part I, Chapter 7. Treatment with perphenazine and with other compounds is described in this and the following Chapter.

Side-effects and complications of the phenothiazines

Patients complain of giddiness when getting up from a sitting position owing to the lowering of the blood pressure. An account is given of the side-effects and dangers of these drugs in Meyler (1960). Common side-effects are meiosis, dry mouth and nasal congestion. If the drug is taken over a long period there is a gain in weight often of considerable proportions. Listlessness is common in the early stages. Jaundice is rare but can be a troublesome complication. It occurs in 1 to 3 per cent of patients. It generally develops 2 to 4 weeks after the beginning of treatment. Liver-function studies show that it is of an obstructive character. The alkaline-phosphatase test is always elevated. The jaundice may last as long as 10 months. Sometimes it clears up even if treatment is continued. Many patients have had laparotomies because the surgeon did not know that they were on chlorpromazine. Every patient with jaundice should be asked about this.

Agranulocytosis which has been fatal with chlorpromazine has not been reported with fentazin or stelazine. The complication can come on as early as 10 days after the beginning of treatment or as late as 400 days. It has occured with as little as 2 grammes of the drug. Two patients who died were having between 600 and 800 mg a day. Another complication is photogenic dermatitis. The patient's appearance is startling. There is a copper colour of the skin and he is oedematous with itching and burning sensations. This photosensitivity can cause keratoconjunctivis (Cahn and Levy, 1957).

There is a definite danger in giving largactil intravenously even if the drug is well diluted and given slowly. There may be a sudden fall of blood pressure which can endanger life. Some patients have an idiosyncrasy for this and a collapse has been known after the administration of only 25 mg by mouth. Decrease of libido can be marked but is generally reversible when the drug is given up.

A serious complication is the reduced resistance to infectious diseases (Gooszen, 1961). A further danger to life is the inability to react to stress through the failure of autonomic reflexes to function adequately such as those connected with raising the blood pressure and increasing cardiac output. For instance patients have died from ECT who were on high doses of largactil, though as much as 150 mg per day can be safely allowed during ECT.

The relationship between the therapeutic effect of phenothiazines and the occurrence of extrapyramidal symptoms

This problem has been discussed by Goldman at the Montreal Conference in 1959 (Goldman, 1960).

For most cases of schizophrenia drugs such as chlorpromazine, fentazin or melleril are sufficient to improve most of the symptoms. However it is sometimes necessary to use a rather more powerful drug such as thioperazine (majeptil) (Delay and Deniker, 1960; Arnold *et al.*, 1960), or fluphenazine (moditen) (Holt and Wright, 1960). These however produce very strong Parkinsonian symptoms. The problem is whether one should diminish the Parkinsonian symptoms by means of an anti-Parkinsonian drug or whether there is a dose level which produces the therapeutic result without the onset of the side-effects. In fact both these methods have been successfully used. An anti-Parkinsonian remedy can be successfully combined with these drugs or a dose can be found where the side-effects are relatively slight.

At the other end of the scale the two drugs which are best known for having a good therapeutic effect while having almost no Parkinsonian symptoms are, as already stated, thioridazine (melleril) and taractan.

Extra pyramidal side-effects: The condition used to be called pseudo-Parkinsonism but there is little reason for the prefix. The autonomic effects are those of salivation, greasy skin, and hypertonus of muscles, especially of the face. There is a typical flexed posture and gait. There can be a typical tremor. However the most distressing symptom is perhaps acathisia or turbulence, where the patient cannot sit still but must always be moving about and generally also has a fine tremor. Another distressing symptom is dystonia of muscles, and especially the face-neck syndrome where there may be oculogyral spasms, torticollis or spasms of the tongue or throat of an alarming character. Other motor symptoms are of a choreiform character. These however are rarer.

Even where these symptoms occur, they are not as a rule serious. They can either be ameliorated by reduction of the dose or else an anti-Parkinsonian drug may be administered.

Relationship of the chemical character of the drug and the production of Parkinsonism

It may be noted that this is not close. Reserpine has a feebler anti-psychotic action than the phenothiazines and yet the Parkinsonian symptoms are more pronounced. It depends a good deal on the inborn constitution of the individual. It is of interest that there are some alkaloids of Rauwolfia which do not produce either Parkinsonism or an anti-psychotic effect.

TABLE IV

DRUG DOSAGE PRODUCING PARKINSONISM
(mg/day)
(By courtesy of the *Revue canadienne de biologie.*)

Drug	Lowest dose producing Parkinsonism	Highest dose (more than 1 patient) without Parkinsonism
Reserpine	2 mg	21.0 mg
Chlorpromazine	25 mg	1500 mg
Triflupromazine	10 mg	600 mg
Prochlorperazine	15 mg	225 mg
Perphenazine	2 mg	96 mg
Trifluperazine	2 mg	75 mg
Fluphenazine	0.5 mg	60 mg
Thioperazine	1 mg	18 mg
Thioridazine	200 mg	900 mg
Proketazine	20 mg	300 mg
Tindal	40 mg	300 mg
R 1625 (Haloperidol)	4 mg	15 mg

The production of Parkinsonian symptoms depends on the radical at position 2 in the phenothiazine ring system. A chlorine or trifluoromethyl radical produces Parkinsonism. Phenergan does not have such side-effects, having no Cl radical at position 2 (Bennett, 1959).

The piperazine side-chain is responsible for a higher anti-psychotic potency. The Parkinsonian symptoms are also more marked, especially those of acathisia and dystonia. Melleril however may produce a slight degree of acathisia and dystonia but not other extra-pyramidal symptoms.

Table IV is taken from Goldman (1960) and shows the lowest dose that produces Parkinsonism in different drugs and the highest dose that has been given without producing Parkinsonism. This list shows how individual differences in the patient are more responsible for the symptoms than the drug itself (see also Ayd, 1960 a).

In the piperazines too which include stelazine, perphenazine and fluphenazine as well as majeptil, the degree of Parkinsonism seems to depend on the radical at position 2. The dimethyl sulphonyl one of majeptil is the strongest and then the trifluoromethyl of fluphenazine and finally the Cl radical of perphenazine.

The two chief compounds which are not phenothiazines but which are used in the treatment of schizophrenia are haloperidol (serenace) and nitoman. The latter resembles serpasil in its pharmacology. According to Goldman the side-effects of haloperidol are rather more difficult to control than those of other drugs.

Goldman has shown that the production of Parkinsonian symptoms is not necessary to effect a remission, because the number of patients discharged without Parkinsonian symptoms are about the same as those who are discharged with them. Nevertheless he considers that majeptil, which produces the most severe Parkinsonian symptoms, is also capable of causing a remission when other phenothiazines have failed.

Delay and Deniker (1960) have also discussed the relationship between the therapeutic effect and the development of Parkinsonism. They were impressed by the fact that majeptil could cause remissions where other phenothiazines had failed. Nevertheless they were cautious in concluding that the Parkinsonian symptoms were necessary for the production of the therapeutic effect.

Freyhan (1961 a) suggests that the therapeutic efficiency of a number of drugs is almost in inverse proportion to the degree in which they produce Parkinsonian symptoms. He found that melleril had the highest therapeutic ratio (0.4) but it also had almost the lowest proportion of Parkinsonian side-effects. On the other hand majeptil had a poor therapeutic ratio (1.13) while fluphenazine, stelazine, fentazin and stemetil were about the same. Vespral was second only to melleril in therapeutic efficiency and vespral also produces Parkinsonism in very few patients. Freyhan's figures do not negative the possibility that majeptil given in the correct dosage is a more powerful drug for chronic schizophrenics than say melleril or vespral which are more successful in moderate cases. The conditions of his treatment were different from those of Goldman.

Baruk and Launay (1961) have used the macac monkey to investigate the physiological effects of chlorpromazine and they distinguish between low dosage which causes psychological effects on the monkey and larger doses which produce neurological effects such as hypertonus, tremors, sweating, etc. They consider that the phenothiazines should be given to patients in doses low enough to produce psychological benefit without extrapyramidal symptoms.

Conclusion: One may surmise from all this that the optimal therapeutic effect may be obtained when the dose is just below the level that is necessary to produce Parkinsonian symptoms. In other cases higher doses are necessary, given in conjunction with an anti-Parkinsonian drug.

Treatment of Parkinsonian symptoms

Procyclidine hydrochloride (kemadrin) and benztropine methane sulphonate (cogentin) are useful anti-Parkinsonian drugs. In a comparative study, Kruse (1960) found procyclidine in a dosage range of 15-30 mg daily to be the drug of choice in the treatment of the acathisia syndrome. This has been confirmed by Paulson (1960) who has also found that paroxysmal dykinesias like fixated vision, oculogyral crises, torsion spasms, speech and swallowing difficulties were controlled within 10 minutes by slow intravenous injection of 5 mg kemadrin. Paulson later also administrered 5 mg kemadrin intramuscularly at the same time and was thus able to prevent relapses in most cases.

Benztropine methane sulphonate is useful in doses of 1 mg twice daily when sialorrhoea is in the foreground.

Another useful drug against Parkinsonism is orphenadrine (disipal) in doses of 50 mg one to three times a day.

Rate of relapse when the drug is withdrawn

Tuteur et al. (1961) studied the female side of a State Hospital in Illinois over a period of 5 years. Therapy with chlorpromazine and reserpine was started while the patients were still in hospital. Tuteur then noticed an improvement in the atmosphere of the wards. There was much less difficulty in the management of these very difficult chronically disturbed patients. He then began to discharge patients and found that they could return to their home life and obtain employment, if the pharmacotherapy was kept up. At first his relapse rate remained lower than that of the State hospital as whole. However, by the end of 5 years it had become about equal. Nevertheless, enough patients had been discharged to reduce the beds by about one-fifth in the unit in which he was working. There was an out-patient clinic available on the premises, and the patients were encouraged to make use of it, even although this often entailed a very long and expensive bus ride. He also attempted to withdraw the drug from some of the patients with the help of giving placebos but 70 per cent of these relapsed. His conclusion was that these drugs enabled patients to return to living in the community but the administration of the drug had to be kept up indefinitely. An important factor was whether the patient was able to return to a home where he was welcomed and received some support.

A second study was that of Else Kris (1961) who worked at a clinic in New York which received patients from various State hospitals. This had the advantage that the clinic was more easily accessible for the patients and that Kris was able to devote all her attention to these out-patients. In other similar studies the work has been done by those still busily working in a State hospital.

She also showed that the response of many mental patients to tranquillising drugs appeared to be sufficiently positive for them to be able to return to their own occupations or to respond favourably to a new training and at the same time develop a satisfying home life. The drug did not appear to bring about adverse side-effects nor to impede the patient at his work or in learning a new occupation. The drug however needed to be continued on an indefinite basis.

A third study was that of Gross et al. (1961) who examined 144 patients who were treated at Springfield Hospital near Baltimore. He organised a project in which patients were paired with controls. There was a double-blind study to see whether the patient for whom the drug was gradually decreased to zero relapsed to a greater extent than another patient matched for age and other qualities who continued with the drug. These patients were predominantly schizophrenic. The average relapse rate per month for the treated patients was 4 per cent but when the drug was withdrawn the monthly relapse rate was 11.7 per cent per month for the entire withdrawal phase and 13 per cent per month for the period during which they finally received a placebo. It was obvious then that withdrawal of the drug greatly increased the likelihood of relapse. The best time to attempt such withdrawal was during the second year of treatment with the drug which was in current use. The placebo was continued for 6 months in cases which did not relapse.

Though not emphasised by the authors one finding was that those who received ECT in addition to the drug were much more likely to remain well after the drug had been withdrawn. This was much more so if the patient received ECT within the 12 months previous to withdrawal of the drug. Those who had received the drug alone had only a 6 per cent survival rate for living outside hospital after the drug was withdrawn. Patients who had received ECT however in the previous year showed a survival rate of 26 per cent for living in the community. Those who had received ECT more than one year before had a 14 per cent survival rate.

It would therefore appear that the combination of ECT with the phenothiazines at some stage does make survival in the community four times more likely. Even if courses of ECT had to be repeated every 12 months or so, the procedure would be well worth while.

Isolation of excited patients

Two different observers have reported that if there is a disturbed patient in the ward, the other patients soon become affected and it may become necessary to increase the dose of chlorpromazine to various patients. Arnold et al. (1960) have reported that if a patient becomes very excited, aggressive or persecuted, then he should be hurried into a side room by a doctor and attendant and these are not allowed to leave the room until the patient has been calmed down by a sedative. This policy has led to the employment of only two-thirds of the previous quantity of the drug used. Folkard (1957) has claimed that refractory behaviour in a mental ward depends on the excited and aggressive behaviour of only a few patients. A tranquil attitude in the ward could be achieved by giving chlorpromazine only to those few patients who are excitable. Sometimes very high doses are required to achieve this result, as Childers (1961) outpoints.

CHAPTER 5

Piperazine Derivatives and Others

Prochlorperazine, perphenazine and chlorproperazine

In 1956 it was found by Broussolle that a drug called prochlorperazine (stemetil), which was commonly used as an anti-emetic, had an action very similar to that of chlorpromazine but was more powerful (Broussolle *et al.*, 1957). This drug was then employed in a number of clinics and soon after trial was made of closely related substances with the same piperazine side-chain and these were also found to be effective. These include perphenazine (trilafon, fentazin) and trifluoperazine (stelazine). Thiopropazate (dartalan) is another member. Recently however more interest has been paid to two members of this group which are thought to be more powerful in causing a remission of schizophrenia and to be successful where other phenothiazines have failed. These are fluphenazine (moditen, permitil, prolixin) and thioperazine (majeptil).

It is usual for a particular clinic to concentrate on one member of the phenothiazine series and the drug which we chose was perphenazine which we have used since its introduction into Great Britain.

Perphenazine (fentazin) is almost twice as potent as stemetil.

Therapeutically it has a wide action. It is particularly useful in paranoid patients but also acts on schizophrenics in much the same way as chlorpromazine. It is more widely used in cases of psychoneurosis. In general medicine it is used to combat nausea, hiccoughing and vertigo.

Side-effects

It is less toxic than chlorpromazine but clinicians should be on the lookout for jaundice or blood dyscrasias, though these are very rare. The occurrence of a sore throat may indicate severe anaemia. The extrapyramidal symptoms are more marked than with chlorpromazine. Sometimes it is necessary to give a drug like cogentin to combat side-effects. As

References p. 221

a rule however it is better to keep to 12–16 mg daily, when such complications are extremely rare. The drug is particularly suitable for outpatient treatments. For institutional patients the drug may be given in higher doses, often 32 mg per day. One of the most troublesome side-effects is the "face-neck" syndrome. In hysterical subjects there may be dystonic symptoms of the muscles of the throat, tongue or lips.

Use of perphenazine in schizophrenia

A large survey carried out by Casey et al. (1960 a) for the Veterans Administration in the U.S.A. showed that 4 phenothiazines produced the same therapeutic results in schizophrenic patients. These were perphenazine, stemetil, stelazine and chlorpromazine. The dose of perphenazine used was a high one, 50 mg daily (see also Cahn and Lehmann, 1957).

Good results have been obtained (Haran 1960) with doses as low as 12 mg daily though 24 and 32 are more commonly employed in institutions. With 16 mg or under Parkinsonian symptoms are rare.

This drug can be combined with ECT in the treatment of schizophrenia. Two techniques have been described in Part I, Chapter 7, for the combined treatment of schizophrenia with ECT and a phenothiazine derivative. The following case demonstrates not only the action of perphenazine on catatonia but also what modern psychiatry and surgery in combination can do for a woman who in a previous generation would have died of a mental disease in the twenties.

It is a case of schizophrenia treated successfully with fentazin.

It was of an Eastern European, a woman aged 30, who had developed schizophrenic symptoms with auditory hallucinations when a prisoner in an enemy country in 1943 after her father had been murdered. She was still hallucinated and deluded. When she arrived in England in 1946 she threw herself in front of a lorry in response to voices and fractured two limbs as well as receiving head injuries. Surgical treatment for the broken limbs was eventually successful but it required a course of ECT, a course of insulin, a leucotomy and a second course of insulin before she recovered sufficiently in a mental hospital to return to work, which she did for several years before relapsing into hearing voices again in 1958. The patient was seen in her own house where she was lying in bed in a state of stupor. She had been in this state for 10 days. The patient was given 8 mg of fentazin three times a day prior to arrangements being made for her admission to hospital. However within 3 days she attended our out-patient department and said that her symptoms had remitted, and in fact she remained well on 16 mg of fentazin daily. She later married and has had a child and at the present time she is able to work as a seamstress at home. She has no hallucinations or delusions. She relapses when she gives up the drug.

As other writers have reported, perphenazine is effective in cases of paranoia. In addition we have had cases of delusions of change of body shape which have disappeared under the effect of this drug.

Haran (1960 gave only 12 mg of perphenazine a day to 31 schizophrenics and there were 31 controls. After a month the pills were switched round and this continued for another month. There was improvement or much improvement in 27 out of 42 male patients with perphenazine and 12 out of 14 female patients. This was an improvement in 70 per cent. He found it especially good in paraphrenic and paranoid patients. In these cases he went up to 32 mg a day. He also found that catatonic cases did well (see also Ayd, 1957).

Perphenazine in depression

We have noticed the energizing and euphoriant effect of this drug. One woman suffering from depression said that the drug gave her a lift, so that she wanted to clean out all her cupboards but it was different from the lift which she had previously experienced with amphetamine, because the latter drug made her tense and anxious at the same time and gave her a hang-over the next day. With perphenazine however the feeling of well-being was less intense but it was accompanied by a feeling of calm. She said that the drug made her want to get out of bed and do something. This effect has been noticed by other workers, especially with the closely allied stelazine (Vogt, 1961). Another patient said that he took amphetamine after breakfast and after his mid-day meal but he took 4 mg of fentazin at 6.00 *p.m.* because it gave him a lift without preventing him from sleeping. By way of contrast with imipramine and some monoamine oxidase inhibitors, the euphoriant effect can occur almost immediately after the drug has been given intramuscularly. The effect on depression was more noticeable if the patients were agitated. If the depression is severe, then it is better for the patient to have ECT and imipramine. It is effective in some cases where there is a mixed psychosis. A man of 65 had suffered for many months from melancholic delusions that his feet and legs were covered with parasites. He was very depressed and had not eaten or slept well but the administration of 12 mg of fentazin a day caused his symptoms to remit. We have found that fentazin was particularly suitable for old patients. As they are more sensitive to the action of any drug, 12 mg daily is enough for them. For hypochondriacal and psychosomatic symptoms, perphenazine acts at least as efficiently as chlorpromazine in blocking the pathway by which the visceral sensations are conveyed to the diencephalon. Perphenazine has a blocking action but it is important that one should distinguish between symptoms which have no organic basis but are in the nature of hallucinations, such as bad smells and bad taste, from those caused by an organic condition such as a tumour of the hippocampal region. Also if an epigastric pain tends to clear up after the administration of perphenazine, one must be sure that the organic condition is improving, and that the drug is not merely acting as an anodyne. A dose of 24 mg a day has greatly relieved two patients of ours who had a very severe pain in the back following an injury. A man who had suffered from very disagreeable hallucinations of smell following a gunshot wound in the head, stated that this symptom cleared up with 24 mg of fentazin daily. We found that in skin conditions patients can be dissuaded from scratching more easily if they are given a daily dose of 8 to 12 mg of fentazin.

We have found that in obsessional illness perphenazine is very helpful in doses of about 16 mg a day but if this is combined with three-quarters of a grain of amytal three times a day, the effect is even more marked. the effect of fentazin on anxiety states is often satisfactory. It acts in some measure through the blocking action of disagreeable and frightening somatic sensations, especially in the head. In addition the euphoriant effect has a favourable influence on the anxiety. The best dose is 12 to 16 mg a day. The blocking action often favours the symptom of frequency of micturition. This ability to hold water longer during the day will help the nocturnal enuresis if that is also present, and 8 mg of perphenazine at night will often reduce the frequency of bed-wetting. Where however the degree of anxiety is very marked and the hypochondriacal symptoms are less noticeable, then the combination of an MAOI with chlordiazepoxide (librium) may be successful (Sargant and Dally, 1962).

In dealing with out-patients it is generally better to start with smaller doses such as 4 mg twice a day. If there are no ill effects one can increase this dose to 12 or 16 mg per day. We found that acathisia and turbulence were very rare unless the dosage reached 24 mg a day. With higher doses we did occasionally have complaints in hysterics of spasms of the muscles of the tongue, lips and throat, and shivering attacks and the feeling that the patient was walking sideways. With 12 to 16 mg a day however there was often a definite euphoriant and calming effect and instead of the patient being restless, there was merely an increase of energy which was often sufficient to make the patient want to return to work, but with larger doses the effects could be the opposite. A patient might want to sleep during the day with 24 mg.

It would seem advisable that outpatients should not have the drug for more than 3 or possibly 6 months unless the case is one of chronic schizophrenia. One patient said that she gave up the drug because she felt she was becoming too dependent on it.

Conclusion

We have described this drug at greater length because it is the phenothiazine which we have used most frequently. It is of especial value in an out-patient clinic. It is useful for those schizophrenics who are living outside an institution, especially those with paranoid symptoms. Its action in combining a euphoriant effect with a sedative effect is of special interest and makes it suitable for the treatment of the more severe psychoneuroses with obsessional symptoms and also some agitated depressions. If however the patient is very depressed or very anxious, other measures may be more successful. We found that the best dosage was about 16 mg daily for the average patient.

The effects of chlorproperazine (stemetil, compazine) are similar (Milne and Fowler, 1960). The dosage is 75-125 mg per day.

Stemetil is one of the drugs by which results have been obtained which are equivalent to those of largactil in an extensive trial organised by the Veterans Association of America for schizophrenics (Casey et al., 1960).

Trifluoperazine (Stelazine)

This is a potent piperazine. Its trifluoromethyl group at position 2 gives it a greater potency than prochlorperazine which has a Cl radical there.

In the higher dosage range, extrapyramidal symptoms are more marked than with chlorpromazine. These side-effects include Parkinsonism, dyskinetic reactions with spasms of the muscles in the face, neck, tongue and throat, and oculogyric crises. Acathisia and motor restlessness are also prominent. However with dosage of 8 mg daily or less, only 2 per cent show such symptoms. Where a high dose is necessary in a mental hospital, cogentin can be used.

Dosage for ambulant patients: often 3 mg daily suffices but up to 6 mg daily may be given.

There have been some favourable reports recently. Stanley and Walton (1961) reported that it was good for moderate cases of schizophrenia. The recovery rate was not influenced by age or type of schizophrenia.

McNeill and Madgwick (1961) compared the effects of stelazine with those of insulin coma. Forty-seven cases treated by stelazine were compared to 63 cases subjected to insulin coma therapy. They were matched for age. With stelazine, 94 per cent improved compared to 75 per cent of the insulin-treated. After 9 months 28 per cent of the stelazine-treated patients were re-admitted but 59 per cent of the insulin patients were re-admitted. Those treated by stelazine were in hospital only 12 weeks but those treated by insulin were in hospital 30 weeks.

Macdonald and Watts (1959) also obtained similar results.

If the drug is given intramuscularly at the beginning of treatment in doses of 1 or 2 mg every 48 hours effects are obtained more quickly.

Thioridazine (melleril)

This drug introduces a piperidine side-chain in place of the aliphatic side-chain of chlorpromazine in position 10 and it has a thiomethyl radical (-SCH) in position 2. The side-chain at position 10 is associated not only with reduced adrenolytic and anti-cholinergic activity but also with suppression of both anti-emetic and extrapyramidal effects. Melleril differs from chlorpromazine in its action on animals. Pharmacologists find that with most phenothiazines, emotionally caused defaecation is prevented about the same level of dosage as that which inhibits a conditioned escape response. With melleril however the escape response persists after the visceral response has been inhibited. Melleril shows a lack of effect on the motor system in other ways. Thus it requires 10 times the dose of melleril to produce catalepsy in mice, in comparison with chlorpromazine, while emotional defaecation is inhibited to a greater degree, as mentioned in Chapter 1 (p. 115). These findings might lead one to predict few Parkinsonism effects but a marked sedative action in man, and this has in fact been found.

Clinical effects

Kinross-Wright (1959) gave a favourable report on 81 schizophrenics who had failed to improve with other methods. In acute cases he claimed 61 per cent "very satisfactory" and in chronic paranoid cases 32 per cent "very satisfactory" results. Remy (1958) reported that in 152 cases there was a total absence of Parkinsonian symptoms and the drug was particularly effective in states of excitement where the patient had made a poor response to previous therapy. The dose ranged from 150 to 400 mg daily. He reported improvement in 78 per cent of schizophrenics.

Sandison et al. (1960) treated 150 patients with melleril over a period of 2 years. The only positive controlled result related to 8 patients receiving melleril who were matched with 7 on a placebo. The improvement with melleril in that small group was significant. They concluded from clinical observations on 150 patients that melleril was superior to all other phenothiazines in its ability to bring about clinical improvement in florid and over-active schizophrenics with the minimum of side-effects. The dosage employed was between 150 mg to 400 mg daily and no important side-effects were reported. However three authors have mentioned impotence in the form of loss of ejaculation (Freyhan, 1961 b).

May et al. (1960) gave very high doses of this drug to a group of patients. They gave between 3200 and 4000 mg daily compared with the maximum of 500 mg given by Sandison.

With the high dosage given by May et al. cases of retinopathy resulted. The condition was characterised by diminution of visual acuity, brownish colouring of vision and impairment of night vision; examination of the fundus disclosed deposits of pigment and several weeks later oedema. To date, this syndrome has not been observed in patients receiving less than 700 mg per day which is 200 mg more than the dose given by Sandison.

Kristanjansen et al. (1962) reported that 61 chronic schizophrenics were treated either with thioridazine or by chlorpromazine for 12 weeks and then the treatments were reversed for 16 weeks and they employed a double blind technique. Extrapyramidal symptoms and skin eruptions were less frequent with thioridazine than with chlorpromazine. One patient had retinopathy with melleril after an average of 560 mg daily for about 2½ years. The total was 482 g. The other side-effects were the same with both drugs. The efficiency of both drugs was the same.

Retinal changes can occur as a side-effect in a number of drugs including the phenothiazines. One of this group, NP 207, was reported by Malitz and Hoch (1956) to cause symptoms indistinguishable from retinitis pigmentosa. Eleven out of 82 patients had some degree of retinopathy. For this reason the drug was never put on the market, these complications having occurred in a preliminary clinical trial.

Ambrosio (1957) made an ophthalmological examination of 220 patients on chlorpromazine therapy. There were two cases of pigment changes which he considered to be unrelated to drug therapy. He does not however say what did cause the retinal changes. The facts suggest that it might be worth while for an ophthalmologist to examine routinely all patients in a mental hospital who are receiving high doses of different drugs. Psychiatrists ought perhaps to be more on the look-out for reports that a patient is bumping into things in the half-light or that he is complaining that everything seems to be brown.

There still seems to be some doubt as to whether retinal changes can occur because of the total amount of a drug taken or merely when the dose exceeds a certain daily level. To be on the safe side it is probably advisable for the patient not to be on a drug for a long time if the drug has been reported to produce retinal changes in high dosage.

Jackson (1961) finds it useful for the aged.

Conclusion

Melleril is a drug of considerable theoretical interest because of its high therapeutic efficiency in the absence of Parkinsonian symptoms. Some reports however do not rate its therapeutic efficiency above that of chlorpromazine. The dosage should never exceed 500 mg a day and it is doubtful if the drug should be administered for a period exceeding 6 or 12 months. The clinician should certainly be aware of the possibility of the patient complaining of indistinct vision in the half-light or a brown colouration of vision. Retinal examinations should be routine.

Chlorprothixene (taractan, truxal)

This drug has excited considerable interest in certain parts of the world, particularly Vienna, where Arnold *et al.* (1960) have advocated its use in schizo-affective states in particular but also in certain states of depression and in the milder conditions of schizophrenia (see also Geller, 1960 and p. 95).

Very varying assessments of its value have been published.

The drug has considerable theoretical importance on account of its resemblance to chlorpromazine structurally and because it is said both to have anti-depressive and anti-schizophrenic effects, while at the same time having fewer side-effects and almost no Parkinsonian features.

It differs from chlorpromazine in that in the central ring instead of having an N atom opposite the S atom, it has a carbon atom which is attached to the same side-chain at position 10 by a double bond. In this respect it resembles amitriptyline. This last drug also substitutes the same carbon atom for the trivalent N atom and has the same side-chain. Amitriptyline however has the same 7-sided central ring as imipramine. Taractan resembles amitriptyline in some respects. It has both an anti-depressant action as well being sedative (Nielsen and Neuhold; 1959).

Taractan resembles chlorpromazine in having the chlorine atom attached at position 2 and in having the same side-chain at position 10.

Pharmacology

Taractan has sedative and adrenolytic properties similar to those of chlorpromazine but it has a greater anti-cholinergic activity. It also has anti-serotonin, anti-histamine, and anti-emetic activity.

When used clinically for treating depression, taractan differs from most anti-depressant drugs in its rapid onset of action. Symptomatic relief, when it occurs, begins to appear within the first day or two of treatment.

Indications and results

It has been used in the more recent and milder forms of schizophrenia, especially those where there is a considerable affective disturbance. It is in this type of case that it has been recommended by Arnold *et al.* (1960).

It has also been advocated for the relief of depression, especially when associated with agitation and anxiety. Feer *et al.* (1960) report the effects of taractan on 88 patients. They gave 120 to 180 mg daily and occasionally 240 mg daily for about 10 days intramuscularly after which they switched over to oral administration of 200 to 400 mg daily. The first reaction was one of marked sedation. Thereafter the patient became very alert and lively and often showed excessive cheerfulness. After the administration had gone on for another 2 or 3 weeks the patient passed into the third phase which was that of more balanced mood and reactions. In schizophrenia the main symptoms affected were motor agitation, volubility and irritability.

The main effect was on endogenous depression, 12 out of 14 such patients showing either improvement or disappearance of symptoms in periods varying from 3 days to 3 weeks.

Poeldinger (1960) described an uncontrolled trial on 102 subjects. The first group was described as consisting of patients suffering from agitation and this included 36 schizophrenics, 1 manic depressive and 12 with organic conditions. He noticed that the effect of taractan was very rapid, taking place within a few hours. It had a marked calming effect and made the use of hypnotics in large doses superfluous. Often hypnotics were not necessary at all, although the patients had been on them for some time. They noted also an euphoriant effect on these patients. He described also 42 cases in which the patient was depressed. This included 6 manic depressives and 21 schizophrenics and 4 with an organic psychosis. They noted again that the action of the drug came on quickly. The results were as follows: in the schizophrenic group 9 out of 21 schizophrenics improved, 5 doing well. This result came on within 5 days. In the organic conditions there were 3 good results and 1 moderate, and out of 11 depressed patients, 5 did well and 4 moderately well. Those that did not respond within 5 days were given other treatment such as ECT. Poeldinger used the same intra-muscular method as Feer *et al.* (1960).

From this pilot study there was a suggestion that the drug had both sedative and anti-depressive effects but that as a neuroleptic it was inferior to chlorpromazine.

Boitelle and Boitelle-Lentulo (1959) had given perhaps the most optimistic account of the drug, finding improvement in 17 out of 18 depressed patients, 11 of these being remissions. Where there was a good response, this occurred within a few days. They claimed that 5 out of 10 hallucinated patients lost their imaginary voices under the influence of the drug. These patients were all paranoid and the other 5 showed some improvement of the paranoia and the hallucinations occurred less frequently. Fourteen schizophrenics showed little benefit from the treatment though agitation was sometimes calmed.

These earlier reports indicated that this drug had a calming and anti-depressive effect but was not primarily indicated in schizophrenia. Later reports tend to confirm this impression although some have denied the anti-depressive effects as well (Bardoni, 1960).

Ravn (1961) had poor results in schizophrenia. Out of 10 hebephrenics there were no cases of marked improvement but 1 of moderate improvement. There were only 7 moderate results in 33 catatonics and in 40 paranoiacs there were 27 moderate results and 1 good result.

The calming effect caused 13 out of 16 manic patients to remit and 1 moderate improvement. He had 34 out of 59 marked improvements in manic-depressive depressed patients, that was 58 per cent remissions and 6, or about 10 per cent, moderate improvement. He had 64 per cent remissions in psychoneurotic depressed states and about 26 per cent moderate results. Only 4 out of 14 anxious patients remitted while 2 were moderate results. He concludes that it is an effective broad range psychotropic agent with a high degree of safety.

Haydu et al. (1961) reported on 47 patients. They gave a dosage of 150 to 300 mg in a day and finally 450 mg a day. They gave it to a succession of patients at a State hospital. The experiment was not controlled. The main symptoms affected were those of excitement. Delusions and hallucinations were the next most frequent symptoms to yield to treatment, then withdrawal and autism, finally depression. Their high dosage led to two cases of leukopenia and one of an increase in the alkaline phosphatase. Somnolence and tachycardia were other side-effects with their high dosage. They concluded that the drug was an effective sedative but that its tranquillising effect was considerably less than that of chlorpromazine and it did not alter delusions or hallucinations. They did not notice any anti-depressant effect of the drug even at high doses.

Darling (1961) carried out a trial in which he matched two groups of 50 patients suffering from retarded or agitated depression. They were matched for age and other qualities. He found that marplan was preferable in cases of non-agitated endogenous depressions but taractan was was superior for agitated depressions. Nearly all the patients required a dose of 30 mg daily of marplan; on the other hand taractan varied between 30 and 400 mg daily. The quiet, unresponsive and listless patient required higher doses of taractan than the agitated patient. Twenty-nine patients improved markedly on marplan and 21 of these were not agitated. Of the 31 patients who improved markedly with taractan 20 were agitated (see also Oltman and Friedman, 1961 a). In 6 involutional psychoses and 24 schizophrenics, Barron et al. (1960) had results inferior to those with stelazine (double blind trial).

Conclusion

Very different results have been reported from different quarters with this drug. This may be due to one or more of several factors. Only one of these was a double blind. Another factor is the report that patients tend to show marked sedation at the beginning of treatment, especially if it is given in high doses intramuscularly. Patients react to the drug in very different ways, some suffering from persistent drowsiness. In most cases the drowsiness gives way to a feeling of excessive cheerfulness. The second phase comes on after about a week. After a second week or so the second phase passes smoothly into a third phase which is characterised by a more normal mood and more normal reactions to the environment. Later observers have not perhaps realised that these reactions succeed each other and hence the varied reports.

The drug appears to have primarily a sedative effect and secondly an anti-depressive effect and thirdly in typical cases of schizophrenia of recent origin good results may be expected. It has even been suggested that racial factors may be responsible for different reactions to the drug.

As so often in modern psychiatric treatment the key to success is a thorough understanding of the therapeutic instrument. It may well be that those who have made a prolonged study of the drug, such as the Vienna group, can obtain results with it which are not achieved by novices. The same holds of majeptil. It requires a long acquaintance with the drug before the clinician can obtain the best results with it.

Fluphenazine (moditen, permitil, prolixin)

The trifluoromethyl radical at position 2 makes the drug more potent than a chlorine atom at that position (stemetil), but less potent than a dimethyl-sulphonyl group (majeptil).

Pharmacology

Because of its greater action in producing hypertonus, it blocks the conditioned avoiding response in rats. It produces hypotension and also tachycardia. Its sedative action is not so marked as in chlorpromazine and it does not potentiate barbiturates.

Side-effects and indications

These are said not to occur if the daily dose does not exceed 1 to 2 mg. They are mostly in the nature of Parkinsonian hypertonus. The dose of 1 mg or 2 mg may be given merely once a day as there is a sustained effect.

Morrow (1961) describes the use of the drug in 174 patients treated on an ambulant basis. They were given doses of 0.5 to 5 mg daily. They were treated up to 2 years. The chief side-effects were wakefulness and Parkinsonian symptoms including "rubber legs". Cogentin was used to combat the extrapyramidal symptoms which occurred in 20 per cent of cases. Her conclusion was that it is a highly effective drug and it is an adjunct to psychotherapy. There were no skin rashes or photosensitivity. There was no liver damage. Acathisia was rare. Patients who had been on other phenothiazines were much more alert when they changed to this drug. It was beneficial in migraine (see also Barsa and Saunders, 1961).

Conclusion

It is probably best to use this drug in comparatively low doses to avoid the extrapyramidal effects. It is a powerful phenothiazine. Its chief interest for psychiatrists up to date has been in relation to the controversy as to whether therapeutic efficiency runs parallel to a drug's tendency to produce Parkinsonian symptoms. In this connection fluphenazine together with thioproperazine (majeptil) have been contrasted repeatedly with the effects of melleril and taractan which produce few extra-pyramidal symptoms. There are not yet sufficient reports to come to a definite conclusion regarding the value of fluphenazine. The drug is not without danger as deaths have occurred which were difficult to explain (Anstreicher, 1960).

Thioperazine (thioproperazine, majeptil)

There has been a definite impression on the part of some experienced investigators that the effects of this drug are more effective in chronic and intractable schizophrenics than some other preparations. At two University Clinics, that of Ste. Anne in Paris under Delay and at the University Clinic of Vienna under Hoff and Arnold, reports have been published in which it has been suggested that this drug is successful where other methods have failed. Denham and Carrick (1961) have published a report in which the clinical observations are very precise and very full. They are convinced that if the patient is kept in a prolonged state of Parkinsonian hypertonus, therapeutic results can be obtained which are very much better than those achieved by other phenothiazines. They report that the patients are often in a state of remarkable suggestibility, so that those who have been resistive and negativistic become unusually obedient and tractable. The suggestibility could also be used to help psychotherapy. These workers state definitely that the degree and extent of muscular hypertonus produced by the drug correlate with the degree of psychiatric improvement.

Denham and Carrick have described the results of their treatment of 60 patients, 42 males and 18 females. With the exception of two manic-depressives all were schizophrenics with an average duration of illness of 10 years. All the patients had previously received some form of medical treatment by one or more neuroleptic agents with little or no benefit. Thirty-two of the 58 schizophrenics achieved total remission of their symptoms after therapy with majeptil. Ten were very much improved, 15 were improved and one was a failure. The two manic patients responded adequately. It was noticed that the patients who had been previously leucotomised appeared to show a less favourable response to thioperazine therapy.

These workers used the so-called discontinuous method of treatment and the average number of courses required in this series was 3.

Technique of discontinuous treatment

Where possible all medication is stopped for a week or two before the beginning of the course. The patient is given 5 mg of the drug three times a day. The drug is gradually increased by 5 to 10 mg thrice daily on alternate days until a dose is reached of about 30 to 50 mg three times a day when it is likely that the continuous state of hypertonus of muscle is reached. Sometimes the dose is raised to 90 mg three times a day. After 5 days of continuous Parkinsonian hypertonus the drug is suddenly withdrawn. The patient is then given a drug-free period of 5 to 7 days by which time all the neurological symptoms will have disappeared. The patient may then be found to have lost his schizophrenic symptoms, in which case a second course may not be necessary. As a rule 3 courses are found to be necessary.

After the maximum therapeutic effect has been obtained, it is advisable to continue the drug on a maintenance basis, which is between 1 and 10 mg daily. Usually one dose a day is sufficient.

Continuous administration

In the method of continuous administration the drug is given at a level which does not produce Parkinsonian symptoms. A suitable starting dose is 5 mg twice or three times a day by mouth. Alternatively about half this quantity can be given i.m. The dose is then gradually increased until the optimum psychiatric improvement is achieved or until neurological symptoms become too troublesome. This level will probably be between 20 and 60 mg daily. If Parkinsonian side-effects should be troublesome, then one can generally reduce the dose or if this is not possible one can give cogentin.

When an adequate psychiatric improvement has been achieved the dosage may then be slowly reduced to a suitable maintenance level.

This drug was the subject of an Annotation in the Lancet (1961) in which these authors' views that the drug removes schizophrenic symptoms by acting on the reticular substance are accepted with caution, as also any suggestion that it is a form of shock treatment.

Attention is also drawn to the fact that failure with previous drugs may have been due to the employment of the wrong dosage or other factors.

In the same journal, Luke and Wyllie (1961) refer to the valuable sedative effect of the drug when given intravenously.

Six months later Cramond (1962) reported that he had been unable to obtain good results by the discontinuous method but he agreed with Luke and Wyllie that it was a valuable drug as a sedative for wildly excited patients when given intramuscularly in a dose of 7.5 mg. Luke and Wyllie gave it in that and even higher dosage.

Conclusion

It is doubtful whether the discontinuous treatment with majeptil forms an exception to the general rule that patients on phenothiazines ought to be kept on a dosage which is below the level at which extrapyramidal symptoms appear. It is not without danger as Annesley and Mant (1962) have described one fatal case.

Haloperidol (serenase)

This is a substituted butyrophenone and was introduced in 1958 by Belgian psychiatrists. In its structure it is comparable to a strong analgesic like pethidine. However it has no analgesic properties but instead it has a marked neuroleptic effect. In animals it inhibits spontaneous activity and conditioned and unconditioned reflexes. Hyperkinetic symptoms are also evident and occur readily.

Indications

Collard (1960) writes that the indications for this drug are paranoid states. These may be expected to respond to treatment either suddenly or gradually within one or two months. Patients with systematic delusions respond better than patients with autistic thinking and fleeting delusions. However the drug strongly inhibits hallucinations in schizophrenia. Haloperidol is also particularly effective for mania, especially for its motor component. Collard claims that the drug is the best non-hypnotic antagonist of agitation from any cause, whether it is endogenous or of extraneous origin, *e.g.* in alcoholism. An intravenous injection of 5 mg inhibits violent agitation in 95 per cent of cases but takes an hour or so to act.

In agitated depression however there is no euphoriant effect but merely a diminution of over-activity.

It is said that there are no toxic effects of this drug on the liver, bone-marrow or skin.

Side-effects

Extrapyramidal symptoms occur in about 80 per cent of cases. Oculogyric crises can be distressing to the patient. In addition, the muscles of the face, neck and tongue may be involved. Parkinsonian symptoms may appear together with rigidity and a mask-like face. Benztropine methane-sulphonate (cogentin) in a dosage of 2 mg twice daily controls the symptoms, or benzhexol hydrochloride (artane) in 5 mg tablets *t.d.s.*

The drug is therefore useful in controlling a wildly manic or excited patient and it may cause the disappearance of terrifying hallucinations.

Oral treatment may be either by high dosage or low dosage. In the former case the patient is given 6 mg daily and this is gradually reduced. Low dosage consists of 0.75 mg daily. After a few days the amount given may be increased to 0.75 mg twice daily and doubled again after a further period. If the drug should be increased, one should wait for a time for the new dosage to take effect before raising it a second time, as it has a long-acting effect. The maintenance dose is between 0.75 and 3 mg daily.

There was a symposium on this drug at Brussels in 1959. The chief finding was that it was useful in controlling very disturbed, excited or manic patients. It was noted that it controlled psychomotor agitation, with only 1.5 per cent of patients developing extrapyramidal symptoms. Delay *et al.* (1960) found the drug very efficient in various psychotic conditions with 3 to 7 mg. It was said to stimulate appetite and increase weight. However, American authors (Azima *et al.*, 1960) and English writers (Garry and Leonard, 1962) have not been enthusiastic. The last named in a controlled trial of 25 chronic schizophrenics matched with 25 controls were unable to send any patients home as a result of the treatment and only 7 improved compared to 4 controls. Brandrup and Krist-jansen (1961) describe a double-blind controlled trial on 36 schizophre-nics. This is the first controlled study published on this drug. Haloperidol produced significantly better results than a placebo.

Conclusion

This drug can be successful in controlling wildly excited or deluded patients. In smaller doses it is suitable for chronic-manic, or hypomanic patients (Samuels, 1961). It is worth trying in schizophrenics who have failed with the less-potent phenothiazine derivatives or in severe schizo-phrenics, especially paranoid patients.

CHAPTER **6**

Non-barbiturate Hypnotics

Although the barbiturates are the most popular hypnotics, it is not uncommon for a therapist to change over to another drug in order to avoid addiction.

Paraldehyde is not popular on account of the taste and because the patient's breath is tainted the next day. Injection of paraldehyde can be painful. Its chief asset is lack of toxicity. It must not be given in a plastic syringe.

Chloral hydrate is an old remedy which is not sufficiently employed today. It is cheap. Its action is certain, prompt and sufficiently lasting and the effects are easily controlled by graduating the dosage. It does not have a cumulative effect. In large doses however it depresses respiration in susceptible individuals, but not if less than 1 gramme is given. The unpleasant taste is its only drawback but that is best masked by syr. zinziber. The old custom of giving it with bromide is unjustified. Dosage 0.3–1.2 g. It is the active principle of welldorm tablets (0.6 g).

Glutethimide (doriden) is probably the non-barbiturate hypnotic which is most used in Great Britain. It takes effect rapidly and has a medium duration of action, comparable to that of amylobarbitone. Sleep may be expected to come on in 20 minutes and last for 6 hours. It is well tolerated and relatively non-toxic. Leucopenia has been reported in a few cases. Dosage: one 250 mg tablet as a sedative, two as a soporific. It should probably not be taken by women of child-bearing age as it has the same nucleus as thalidomide.

Methyprylone (noludar) is effective in moderate cases of insomnia in tablets of 200 mg, and in more severe cases it may be combined with barbiturates. In milder cases, doses of 50 mg suffice. There is no alteration in the blood picture even after prolonged administration.

References p. 221

Methaqualone hydrochloride (melsedin)

The accompanying figure (see appendix) shows the chemical formula which is 2-methyl-3-orthotolyl-4-quinazolone hydrochloride. This drug was originally used against malaria but was not found to be effective. However the experimental subjects were found to fall asleep. The drug was therefore tried out as a hypnotic. It is provided in tablets of 150 mg. The usual dose is 2 at night, and 150 mg has the same effect as 200 mg of cyclobarbitone. A controlled trial showed that both these drugs were superior to a placebo when given in doses of 150 mg and 200 mg respectively. Generally, twice this dose is indicated for sleep. The hypnotic effects were first described in 1955. The drug takes 10 to 20 min to take effect and the sleep lasts for 6 to 8 hours. In the morning there is no dizziness, headache or drowsiness in the great majority of cases.

Pharmacology: It is a more potent hypnotic than phenobarbitone or allobarbitone, but with a much greater margin of safety. It is a more potent anti-convulsant in animals than either phenobarbitone or phenytoin sodium. The action of the drug is potentiated by phenobarbitone, methylpentynol, chlorpromazine or codeine.

The hypnotic effect is never preceded by a state of excitement. The drug depresses polysynaptic reflex arcs in doses which do not inhibit monosynaptic reflexes, spinal ganglia, myoneural junctions or skeletal muscle. It also relaxes smooth muscle and has a weak anti-histaminic effect. It is not however analgesic.

Side-effects: A few patients are resistant to even 300 mg and instead of sleeping react with confusion and headache. There is slight dyspepsia in a few cases. It is used with success for alcoholics.

We have tried it out and have found that it is especially safe. One of our patients took 12 pills in a day and was hardly any the worse, and a single dose of 6 grammes has been reported without permanent ill-effects. Up to the present there has been no evidence of habituation or addiction.

We had one patient, a married woman of 33 who before coming to us had made 22 suicidal attempts by over-doses of barbiturates. On numerous occasions she had taken 90 grains (6 grammes) of amylobarbitone in a day. She had spent three years in a mental hospital on account of addiction.

She made a complete recovery. She has now been well for six months. Part of the treatment was to give her melsedin, which helped her during the withdrawal stages but she did not become an addict to melsedin. She occasionally takes a couple of melsedins at night to sleep. In this case however the main treatment consisted of psychotherapy and hypnosis.

Conclusion: This drug is an extremely useful agent for treating insomnia of mild degree and can be given with safety in doses of up to 600 mg. The toxicity is very low. It is extremely useful in the treatment of drug addicts and alcoholics (Baird and Buckler, 1962).

Methylpentynol (oblivon)

Pharmacology: Although animal experiments indicate a wide margin of safety, nevertheless death in man has been recorded from a dose of 5 grammes. With high doses exfoliative dermatitis may occur. In therapeutic doses there are seldom side-effects though it may produce belching with an unpleasant taste. It potentiates the action of barbiturates and alcohol. It should probably not be given over a long period.

Indications: The drug is used as a hypnotic for nervous patients as it diminishes their anxiety. It can be given with a barbiturate the action of which it potentiates. It produces no hang-over. It can be used for the relief of mild anxiety states and to tide over periods of emotional stress. It is given in capsules of 250 mg or as an elixir, 250 mg per 4 ml, and, as the carbonate, in tablets of 100 mg.

Thalidomide (softenon, distaval): dangers

This drug was used as a sedative and anti-emetic but was found to cause malformation of the foetus in some pregnant women and was withdrawn from the market (Lancet, 1962). This disaster has caused a public outcry with a demand that all drugs should be thoroughly tested before being put on the market. Medical men should certainly advise all married women of child-bearing age to avoid new drugs the effects of which have not been fully investigated.

References p. 221

CHAPTER 7

Tranquillisers or Relaxants

The word tranquilliser is used in English to designate a class of drugs which have a sedative action without being hypnotic. They are distinguished from the neuroleptics which are used predominantly to influence psychotic states. They are given in rather smaller doses than neuroleptics. They may be prescribed to reduce muscular tonus or more commonly to combat anxiety. They can be divided into three main groups (see appendix).

Diphenylmethane derivatives

Benactyzine

These drugs are related to well-known spasmolytic drugs such as adiphenine (trasentin). The tranquilliser benactyzine differs from adiphenine in possessing a hydroxyl group in place of an H-atom. The tranquilliser hydroxyzine bears a close resemblance to the anti-histamine chlorcyclizine (histantin) and meclozine (ancolan).

Most of these compounds have marked anti-histaminic properties. They also possess some atropine-like action and antagonise some of the effects of serotonin. They prolong the action of barbiturates and other hypnotics. In animals they do not produce sedation or have a soporific effect but they can produce convulsions when given in sufficiently high doses. They do not block conditioning but may facilitate it. The main members of this group are azacyclonal (frenquel), benactyzine (suavitil), hydroxyzine (atarax) and phenyltoloxamine (PRN) (Taeschler and Schlager, 1962).

Azacyclonal

Azacyclonal, known as frenquel is given in doses of 20 to 60 mg daily. Its chemical formula is shown in the appendix. It was introduced by Fabing and Hawkins (1956). They had noticed its action in abolishing the effects of psychotogenic drugs, such as LSD and mescalin, and in terminating the EEG changes caused by these drugs. Fabing and Hawkins reported that 5 out of 14 patients with acute schizophrenia lost their symptoms within 1 to 3 days. They said that 12 out of 14 returned to work on maintenance doses and there were no recurrences in up to 11 months. They also recommended it in alcoholic psychosis. They gave high dosage such as 100 mg intravenously followed by 100 mg thrice daily by mouth for at least a week, with progressive reduction of the dosage and withdrawal at the end of three weeks. They did not notice any side reactions. Rinaldi *et al.* (1955) reported in a controlled clinical trial that there was definite improvement in 39 chronic disturbed patients by comparison with the placebo, but relapse followed withdrawal of frenquel. Hargreaves (1959) however in a double blind trial in schizophrenics found it of no value and there was no obvious anti-hallucinatory action. This confirms that the LSD model psychosis is more like a toxic psychosis than schizophrenia.

Indications: It is said to counteract visual hallucinations. It does not cause drowsiness. It does however prolong the action of barbiturates. It has an antagonistic action to the psychomotor stimulant effects of pipradol of which it is a congener. No definite contra-indications are known at present. Clinical trials do not put it in the same class as chlorpromazine for the treatment of schizophrenia. It may be of use in a toxic psychosis and in some aggressive and agitated states.

Conclusion: This drug has not borne out the high hopes which attended its first use. One of its chief virtues is its low toxicity and the absence of side-effects but on the other hand, it is effective only in more acute and relatively mild conditions in which there is restlessness, aggression and possibly visual hallucinations.

Hydroxyzine hydrochloride (atarax)

We prefer atarax to benactyzine. This drug has anti-histaminic and anti-spasmodic actions but its effect as a centrally acting sedative is more marked than some of its congeners. It is employed in the treatment of anxiety and tension states but not in depression or the psychoses. It is used to control ventricular arrhythmia. It is however doubtful whether this action is superior to that of mild barbiturates. It is probably inferior in this respect to quinidine.

Perhaps its chief indication is for skin diseases as it certainly prevents or diminishes the patient's inclination to scratch in such diseases of chronic urticaria. Its anti-secretory function may diminish the amount of sebum secreted in some cases of dermatitis. In cases of dyspepsia it is likely to diminish gastric secretions and counteract any tendency to colic.

It has a low toxicity. There can be a slight drowsiness when it is first given but this does not promote sleep and passes off even when the drug is continued. The drug increases the tendency to bleed in patients receiving anti-coagulant therapy. It potentiates the action of barbiturates. The usual dose is 25 to 100 mg *t.d.s.* It can be given i.m. in doses of 50 to 100 mg every 4 to 6 hours while an i.v. dose of 50 mg may be given initially. It should be given slowly at the rate of 25 mg per minute.

Hydroxyzine pamoate (vistaril)

This drug has a similar action: it is a central nervous system depressant with a local anaesthetic effect. It protects the heart against arrhythmia caused by adrenaline. It antagonises apomorphine. It has an anti-histaminic action.

Indications: It is used for the symptomatic treatment of anxiety and tension. It is useful in psychosomatic disorders, and it is given also for peptic ulcers.

Side-effects: These are mild but again there is temporary drowsiness. Patients complain of paraesthesiae, a feeling of numbness and light-headedness. The usual dose is 25 to 100 mg *t.d.s.* Beckman (1961) gives an account of the literature.

Phenyltoloxamine (PRN)

This drug has been used as a mild sedative for anxious patients.

Pharmacology: Its action is similar to that of the last named drugs. It has an anti-histaminic effect and acts as a depressant on the autonomic nervous system and in higher doses on the central nervous system. It has mild anti-spasmodic properties as well as a local anaesthetic effect. Despite its sedative action it has no adverse effect on mental acuity.

Indications for use: It is used again against anxiety and in skin disorders.

Side-effects: It has a greater tendency to produce somnolence than its congeners. It produces dryness of the mouth, constipation, blurring of vision, heartburn, ataxia, and slight impairment of psychomotor activity. The ataxia is more pronounced in older patients. The usual dose is between 50 and 200 mg three times a day. Its action is described by Conn (1961).

It may be remarked in conclusion that the anti-histaminic which is most widely used for its central sedative action is still promethazine (phenergan, see appendix). It is a suitable antidote for apomorphine given i.m.

Propanediol derivatives

The second group of tranquillisers are those known as the substituted propanediols. From a strictly chemical point of view these compounds are really modified glycols, as they possess two hydroxyl groups attached to different carbon atoms. All members of this group have been evolved from the muscle relaxant mephenesin (Berger and Bradley, 1946). It was noticed that mephenesin, in addition to its relaxing properties, relieved anxiety and nervousness, and chemical modifications of the molecule were carried out to produce compounds that would be better tolerated and would have a more intense and a longer duration of action.

These compounds do not affect the functioning of the autonomic nervous system and in this way they differ from the phenothiazines and from reserpine and from the diphenylmethanes.

They relieve muscle spasms by decreasing conductivity along interneuronal pathways. On the Continent they are called interneurone blockers. As mentioned previously they scarcely affect monosynaptic reflexes. They raise the convulsive threshold to electrical and chemical stimulation. They do not affect conditioned reflexes. They do not appear in usual doses to affect motor performance, reaction time, and other tests requiring judgment and skills (see Uhr and Miller 1960, Chapters 22, 26 and 51). The best known member of this group is meprobamate. This drug raises the frustration threshold and permits performance of behavioural tasks under stress conditions (Holliday *et al.*, 1958).

Meprobamate (equanil, miltown, mepavlon)

Before the advent of librium this drug was perhaps the most popular tranquilliser, especially in the U.S.A.

Clinical effects: It has only a mild hypnotic action, but by its relaxing and tranquillising effects it induces a natural sleep. It has a greater anti-convulsant property than mephenesin from which it is derived. Some patients show a certain drowsiness and the drug causes a slowing of the frequency of cortical rhythm with an increase of voltage in the EEG. It is employed for anxiety in neurotic patients .In larger doses it produces ataxia rather than sleep.

Indication: This drug has a high index of safety. It has been used for petit mal but its main use is in tension states. It is not so successful in treating agitated or depressed patients as librium. It has been much used in the treatment of alcoholism. If used over a long period however patients can become addicted to it as also to the diphenylmethane derivatives.

Side-effects: In high doses incoordination can occur and patients complain of drowsiness and lassitude. Occasionally there are skin troubles such as urticaria and erythema. Acute purpura has been reported.

Paradoxical excitement can occur. Occasional fatalities have been reported (La Verne, 1961 a and b). These are due to idiosyncrasy even at therapeutic level. Where suicidal attempts have occurred there have been coma, absence of deep tendon reflexes, marked relaxation with fixed dilated pupils, shock and hypotension.

This drug has had its champions as well as its detractors. Rickels *et al.* (1959) in testing out the effects of amylobarbitone, stemetil and a placebo, as well as meprobamate in acutely ill neurotic out-patients found that meprobamate was the drug which obtained the best results. Patients suffering from irritability, mild depression and insomnia were said to be relieved. On the other hand, Moriarty (1959) did not find the drug superior to a placebo. Batterman *et al.* (1959) found it no better than the barbiturates given in small doses.

The consensus of opinion is that meprobamate is of use mostly in anxiety states of recent origin where the symptoms, especially hysterical ones, are not marked.

The fact that addiction can occur makes it unsuitable for administration over an unlimited period (Essig and Ainslie, 1957).

Phenaglycodol (ultran)

This is a mild depressant for the central nervous system. It does not dull mental acuity. The general opinion is that this drug is less effective than the closely related meprobamate. More facts are required before it can be accepted as an effective agent. It is contra-indicated in depression and if the patient takes an overdose there may be coma and respiratory arrest. The patient ought to be under medical supervision (Zukin *et al.*, 1959).

Conclusion: Drugs of this class act in a manner which in some ways resembles the effects of small doses of barbiturates. Both classes of drug inhibit the polysynaptic reflexes, such as the bending and stretching reflex, and they also have an anti-convulsive effect, whether the convulsion is caused by cardiazol, strychnine or electroshock. In higher doses meprobamate causes motor incoordination and ataxia. In mice meprobamate causes an increased activity in doses which are not quite high enough to produce incoordination. It also increases the amount of food consumed. With lower doses there are many parallels between the actions of these two groups, but in higher doses the actions are different. A typical tranquilliser does not cause sleep even in fairly high doses, whereas the barbiturates do so.

Diazepines

There is also a third class of tranquillizer, the diazepines with a similar action to that of meprobamate. Librium is the best known of this group.

Chlordiazepoxide (librium)

This drug has an action very similar to that of meprobamate, but in some ways it is more potent. The diazepines contain a ring system with 7 atoms, two of which are N atoms. In this respect they resemble imipramine (tofranil). Amitriptyline also has a 7-sided ring but has no nitrogen atom in it. It is of interest that chlordiazepoxide also has some anti-depressive effects as well as being probably the most successful tranquillizer to date. Its anti-depressive action appears to be stronger than that of meprobamate. Librium has an anti-convulsive action and it causes ataxia in higher doses (see appendix).

Clinically it is not only highly potent in the treatment of neurotic patients suffering from anxiety and tension but it is also effective to some degree in combating depression and the agitation which accompanies melancholia. It thus combines a sedative action with a euphoriant action.

It has been recommended in the following conditions: anxiety neurosis, tension, headaches, pre- and postmenstrual tension, chronic alcoholism, agitated depression, acute agitation, hysterical or panic states. More recently it has been tried in the acute stages of schizophrenia. It is useful both for children and old people. In the latter case, as with children, the dose is smaller.

Sargant and Dally (1962) combine it with phenelzine in affective disorders that might be described as reactive depressions but which include hysterical phobic and anxiety symptoms. We have also found that it combines very well with imipramine in the treatment of agitated depression either where ECT has been given or not. Tobin *et al.* (1960) are enthusiastic about its effects in mild depressions and in anxiety states. Patients who suffer from phobic, obsessional, compulsive, depressive, tense and lethargic states, and those with conversion symptoms and hysterical acting-out did very well. These workers claimed 18 per cent excellent results and another 27 per cent good results, with 19 per cent fair results. One effect which we noticed and which is mentioned by Jenner *et al.* (1961) is that patients who receive 30 mg during the day, state that a sleeping pill is no longer necessary. The action may be compared to that of a new drug called dipiperon, or R 3345. This is a neuroleptic drug described by Bobon and Collard (1962). This drug is a butyrophenon. The title of their paper was "Dipiperon, a new neuro-leptic with a delayed hypnogenic effect". They reported that the administration of this drug by day facilitated in a remarkable manner the onset of sleep at night without causing any somnolence during the day. The duration of sleep was facilitated in 85 per cent of cases and the depth of sleep in 88 per cent and the time taken to fall asleep was shortened in 91 per cent. Those whose sleep improved remained normal in 45 per cent of cases. This new idea in psychiatry is worthy of note. Dipiperon is related to haloperidol.

Kinross-Wright *et al.* (1960) described the effects of librium on 136 patients. They received 10 to 40 mg daily (30 mg daily is considered the optimum). Out of 19 neurotics there was 67 per cent improvement. The predominant effect was a reduction of anxiety, agitation and aggression. There was also elevation of affect; the patients became less restless and were able to socialise their over-activity. If doses of over 50 mg daily were given, drowsiness and ataxia could be observed.

The British Medical Journal (1960) in a review of the actions and uses of the drug states that in some patients obsessional symptoms and tension have been made worse. This is certainly not our experience. It is always necessary to ascertain what the correct dosage is for each drug. Some unfavourable reports result from too high a dose being given to patients and then the side-effects complicate evaluation of the drug. In this instance rather higher doses were given at first, whereas with some other drugs the value has been underestimated because of too little being given. The article continues to say that there is no place for it in the treatment of schizophrenia, which is in fact now doubtful. Bambace (1961) has reported favourably on a series of 73 outpatients treated with this drug. In most of the patients who were psychotic, phenothiazine therapy had been administered, but the results were said to be unpredictable partly on account of side-effects. The patients were therefore switched over to librium because of its freedom from complications. About a third of the patients were schizophrenic while the other two-thirds were either neurotic or had personality disorders. The average dose was 30 mg a day and they were treated up to 6 months. Seventy-five per cent of the patients were said to show good or excellent results. The best response was in the psychoneurotic group where there were 17 out of 21 good results, and 6 out of 7 other patients diagnosed as anxiety reaction also did well. Two mentally deficient patients were improved. Eleven out of 25 schizophrenics showed an excellent response and 4 a good response. The drug was not found to be of use in either paranoid or manic-depressive patients.

Jenner *et al.* (1961) in a controlled study of 92 patients concluded that librium was likely to be superior to amylobarbitone for the symptomatic relief of a neurotic patient. They used 60 mg a day, which they later considered to have been to high. They recommend 30 mg a day. They remark on the safety of the drug. Hines (1960) has reported that a schizophrenic female aged 47 took 1,150 mg of librium in 20 minutes while a male patient of 22 took 1,600 mg in 24 hours. In neither case was gastric lavage used and no long term physical impairment was caused. In contrast, barbiturates are one of the commonest suicidal agents. They had the impression that although barbiturates may lose their effect owing to habituation, this would probably not be so if it were combined with librium. They state that for out-patients librium appears to be superior to amylobarbitone.

Schopbach (1961) also reports favourably on this drug. He describes 53 consecutive patients in an out-patient clinic. Librium was beneficial in 60 per cent of obsessional compulsive patients and for about one-third of others suffering from chronic neuroses or depression. These benefits achieved by patients previously considered unpromising, indicate that this drug is a valuable addition to our armamentarium. He gave 10 mg *q.d.s.* and found side-effects minimal. This study however was uncontrolled and the numbers were small.

Side-effects: These are negligible in doses of 30 or 40 mg daily. With high doses one obtains ataxia, drowsiness, skin rashes, nausea, constipation, increased or decreased libido. Paradoxical reactions such as excitement, stimulation, acute rage and elevation of affect, have all been reported. The appetite is stimulated and the patient gains weight. The blood pressure can be slightly reduced. Slurred speech, tachycardia, palpitation and flatulence have all been reported.

There are now indications that patients are beginning to misuse the drug. It is not unusual for psychopathic patients to take 120 mg a day regularly. It has occurred frequently in the history of a drug that a report is made that there are no symptoms of addiction, but it always takes a few years before they are recognised. It would therefore appear unwise to give this drug for more than a few months at a time.

Abrupt cessation of medication produces withdrawal symptoms in a high proportion of cases. It is similar to withdrawal of barbiturates and even convulsions have been reported. Elderly patients should receive capsules of only 5 mg. Patients should be warned not to take it if they are driving a car or if they are engaged in work that requires manual dexterity (Hollister *et al.*, 1961).

Conclusion: It seems likely that despite an uncertain beginning both in America and in England, this drug will prove to be one of the most valuable of the tranquillisers.

References p. 221

CHAPTER 8

Abreactive and Psycholytic Drugs

Psychiatrists working under the National Health Service still aim at finding a method of psychotherapy which will be as effective as psycho-analysis at its best but which will not take so much time. Freud (1933) wrote of the need to use chemical agents to assist "psychological levers" in coping with the powerful psychological forces at work in certain psychiatric conditions. Horsley was the first to write on what he called narco-analysis (Horsley, 1936). He used intravenous barbiturates not only in the neuroses but also for cases of catatonia. He also used such methods for the war neuroses, as also did Sargant and Shorvon (1945).

We have generally preferred to use a combination of sodium amylo-barbitone intravenously in combination with methedrine. These are given from different syringes but through the same needle. The dose is about 150 to 300 mg of the barbiturate, preferably in 2.5 per cent solution and about 5 to 15 mg of methedrine.

Some workers have used methedrine and more recently ritalin alone but most psychiatrists believe that on the principle of one's first duty being not to harm the patient, large doses of methedrine or ritalin alone intravenously is a little risky. In any case the patient may take two or three hours to recover from such high doses.

Indications

Narco-analysis is very useful in psychosomatic complaints. Even the most severe case of psychogenic vomiting or tachycardia can generally be im-proved by this procedure.

In the out-patient department of a general hospital it is not uncommon for a patient to be admitted with loss of memory. Many of these subjects however are in trouble with the law. Others are trying to escape from a difficult environment. Some may remain too drowsy when given sodium amytal alone, but its combination with methedrine loosens the tongue much better. One of our patients said that he had resisted the effects of sodium amytal easily at a previous hospital but was compelled to speak when given the two drugs in combination.

The various methods of narco-analysis can be compared, with regard to certain drawbacks. One should consider whether apparatus is required, whether the induction of the relaxed state can be brought about easily, and whether the patient will require attention over a period of an hour or more and whether any serious side-effects are to be anticipated. Another problem is whether staff are needed and whether the treatment is expensive. Sodium amytal and methedrine in combination avoid many of the disadvantages mentioned. Good effects can be brought about easily in a large proportion of patients. It is only a small number who may become more depressed. A schizophrenic who has escaped diagnosis may become worse owing to methedrine. This drug is contraindicated, if there is a suspicion of schizophrenia as he may become excited.

In most cases an increased rapport between the patient and the physician develops and the former can talk easily and with considerable emotion about his problems.

The patient is often in a highly suggestible state, and with a barbiturate alone a state of hypnosis with suggestion can often be induced. Massion Verniory caused the progressive disappearance of a painful phantom leg by means of suggestion under intravenous thiopentone in successive sessions (personal communication).

We have found this method good for treating the patient whose sexual conditioning is abnormal. Such a patient can talk easily about the incidents in his psychosexual development which have had an importance in leading to the deviation.

The word psychosynthesis has been used to describe the building up of the patient after his inhibitions have been broken down. The patient has a strong urge after the recovery of lost memories to develop a new positive attitude towards his environment.

As we shall see, there have been some doubts about the ultimate good effects of this type of treatment compared with conservative measures. However there are always some cases which the therapist feels sure would not have recovered but for energetic treatment of this kind.

Narcoanalysis has its limitations and the results in treating chronic obsessional illness are often disappointing. In the experience of many psychiatrists the repeated bringing into consciousness of emotionally charged material in obsessionals has a beneficial effect, which however is only temporary. Often the physician tries to bring the material up again and produce another abreaction. However he fails in this and the long-term results of psychotherapy in obsessional illness are known to be poor. This is what justifies the use of the new psychopharmacological approach.

When it has been necessary to abreact some war experience or other terrifying event we have preferred to use subconvulsive electrical stimulation, making sure that the current was sufficient to penetrate the brain. As already mentioned, this method produces the strongest degree of mental dissociation and the patient relives his past experiences in the most dramatic manner. In that technique we used "noises off- stage". The imitation of the sounds of a machine gun or those of exploding bombs could cause the most violent abreaction. A patient could continue for an hour or more in a state of somnambulism.

The results of this treatment are different from those of amytal and methedrine, since much stronger reactions can be obtained by it.

The use of carbon dioxide therapy

This was introduced by Meduna in 1946 (Meduna, 1950), for the treatment of the psychoneuroses. It was found not to be beneficial in cases of schizophrenia. The treatment can be quite alarming for the patient and side-effects of an unpleasant character can occur. One of our patients, a hysteric, complained of paralysis of the legs after treatment. However in most cases there is a feeling of excitement followed by relaxation and a feeling of well-being. Not uncommonly a so-called CO_2 dream occurs but the experience has some differences from a typical dream. It is more like looking at a static picture or cartoon of one's life situation at the moment. Sometimes the effects are striking. A homosexual schizoid patient of ours after treatment had a sudden change over to a heterosexual attitude. On the first attempt at coitus his genitals were completely anaesthetic during the experience but on the second attempt the sexual experience was natural. Although he had had insulin coma and ECT, he said that CO_2 was much the most beneficial and frequently asked that it be repeated.

A curious fact is that the treatment can be given to the patient when he is standing up as CO_2 increases muscle tone. The procedure can be associated with a specific type of psychotherapy, which was developed by Wilcox (1951). The patient has a so-called dream under the CO_2, and can discuss it when he awakes, and the fact that the psychiatrist is in close contact with the patient's unconscious leads to curious but effective conversations. It is an interesting experience to witness Wilcox's technique.

Although the usual technique is for the patient to take 30 to 40 respirations of 20 per cent CO_2 in oxygen (and this produces a state of coma) in other cases the psychiatrist keeps the patient just under the dose which produces a coma. In this way he often obtains material which has been repressed and which is of great significance for psychotherapy.

Meduna himself has stated that psychotherapy is not necessary but he believed that the inhibitions of cortical function and the release of the sub-cortical centres from its control had a beneficial effect on the patient. From our experience we would say that as with sub-convulsive electrical stimulation, active psychotherapy is an essential part of treatment.

Tibbetts and Hawkings (1956) have carried out a trial on patients half of whom received CO_2 treatment and the others the same treatment except that compressed air was used instead of the CO_2. They stated that the results were about the same in both cases; the number of patients who were much benefited was in the nature of 50 per cent. CO_2 has now largely been abandoned for the treatment of the neuroses. However as with other therapies if the psychiatrist is skilled in its administration then the therapeutic effect may be very good.

Ether

This was used in the war for patients who were either grossly inhibited because of some hysterical reaction or because of a panic state. Sargant and Slater (1954), reported that if a state of excitement was followed by the sudden onset of complete exhaustion and collapse, the patient was likely to show a good result from the treatment. Ether however has become almost completely abandoned to-day for narco-analytic purposes partly because of the difficulties of giving the treatment which must be carried out in hospital. As with nitrous oxide patients sometimes have a

References p. 221

curious experience. They feel that they have suddenly come to understand the "secret of the universe", but unfortunately the secret eludes them when they wake up again! Some have even asked to have the experience a second time to recapture the illusion.

Lysergic acid diethylamide (LSD)

LSD-25 is a synthetic amide of *d*-lysergic acid with a secondary amine, and belongs to the ergonovine group of ergot alkaloids. It is the best known member the psychotomimetic group of drugs which can produce a "model psychosis" with characteristic hallucinogenic and usually mild stimulant properties.

In experimental psychiatry LSD has a firmly established position; hundreds of articles attest to the growing interest in its psychotomimetic activity. As an adjunct to psychotherapy however its potential has not yet been completely investigated.

The drug has been administered to normal subjects and used in almost every known psychiatric disorder.

Stoll (1949), who reported in detail the chemistry and pharmacology of the drug, considered that the symptoms produced by LSD-25 in the normal subject were an expression of an acute endogenous psychosis analogous to that produced by alcohol, opium, cocaine, hashish, mescaline or the amphetamines. There is no uniform reaction to LSD-25, a fact that gives it a special interest, although Becker (1949), and some others have distinguished two main types — (a) manic or depressive reactions, and (b) schizophrenic reactions; the majority of subjects showed a mixture of these two extreme types. The studies in normal subjects which have also been reported on by Condrau (1949), Fischer *et al.* (1951) and Matéfi (1952) have enabled a great deal of material to be collected from which the probable behaviour of psychoneurotic patients might be predicted.

The effects of LSD on psychotic patients have been reported by Stoll (1947), Busch and Johnson (1950), De Giacomo (1951), Condrau (1949) and others. Psychotic changes in these patients, however, can only be found after large doses and take the form of an exaggeration of the psychotic state.

Busch and Johnson (1950) reported their results after giving LSD-25

to 8 cases of psychoneurosis. The drug was used as an aid to psychotherapy and all patients had experiences which profoundly influenced
the course of their illness.

Physiological effects

Most of the physiological effects of LSD are mediated through the autonomic nervous system, the majority being sympatho-mimetic in nature.
There is dilatation of the pupils, sweating, flushing, anorexia, nausea and
occasional vomiting; deep tendon reflexes are accentuated. Blood pressure
is usually increased. There can be initial giggling and laughing as in
hypnosis. Changes found in the electroencephalogram are disappointingly
few, the only consistent finding being an increase of 1—3 c/s in the alpha
rhythm (Abramson, 1957; Busch and Johnson, 1950; Cohen et al. 1958).
Some form of dysarthria may be demonstrated in approximately 30 per
cent of those taking the drug (Condrau, 1949). One effect is that the
adrenal cortex is less responsive to ACTH. It decreases urinary phos-
phatic excretion, but markedly increases it after stimulation by ACTH.

Psychological

By and large the LSD experience is a pleasurable one, but even stable
individuals sometimes experience an unpleasant and terrifying one.
Several psychoses have been precipitated, some with suicidal inclinations,
particularly in predisposed individuals, while occasionally some particularly undesirable effects of the drug last for several days. These complications have been well summarised by Cohen (1960).

Certain factors have affected the reactions: decreased amount of food
or sleep results sometimes in a severe reaction. Personality is also of
importance, while if the patient is distracted during the reaction the
latter is probably less effective. Solitude seems to increase the severity of
the reaction. The milieu and the mental environment of the patient is
important, a psychiatrist deriving more from the experience than a lay-
man, while the patient is eager to please his psychiatrist.

Course of events

The effects of the drug depend on the method of administration. It can be given either by mouth or by intra-muscular or intravenous injection. The intravenous route produces the quickest response, then the intra-muscular and last the oral. Depending on the method of administration, the prodromal effects begin approximately after ten to twenty minutes and last about one and half hours, consisting primarily of autonomic changes and associated symptoms. The height of the reaction occurs from two to four hours after the ingestion and the end of the reaction varies from five to twelve hours. During this period there is usually reduced activity, though not in all cases; also poverty of thought, indifference, and shallow affect. After-effects of the drug may last from one to several days, with subdued behaviour, occasional irritability and frequently increased introspection (Sandison, 1954).

Perceptual anomalies

Perceptual anomalies predominate and there is increase of visual imagery. With eyes closed and in a darkened room, a variety of lights, flowers, bursting bombs and a very wide variety of complexity in patterns are observed. There are frequently complex hallucinations. Occasionally frightening images are noticed and some individuals report movements on the walls as if the room were breathing in and out.

Auditory hallucinations are seldom observed, although hyperacusis is very common.

There is frequently an alteration of body image and distortion of feeling, with anaesthesia or hypoanaesthesia present. Time and space are usually distorted and ego sense is disturbed. (Hoch, 1959).

The patient frequently projects on to the environment and will identify the therapist with parents or others close to him, either as kindly or frightening punitive figures. Suspiciousness directed towards the therapist it not uncommon. Under the influence of LSD the subject retains insight at all times and is aware that he has taken a drug and is participating in an experience. Alteration of consciousness is rarely seen but poverty of thought, impairment of abstract thinking, indecision and distractability often manifest themselves. Wechsler Bellevue studies reveal that LSD disturbs concentration, impairs contact with the environment and generally reduces intellectual functioning.

The drug has been considered to produce a schizophrenic-like response, but there is now considerable evidence after some years of controlled observation to indicate that the LSD phenomena are dissimilar to schizophrenic characteristics (Condrau, 1949). These are: Visual perceptual distortions under LSD-25 are almost never seen in schizophrenia; visual hallucinations are characteristic of the LSD experience, while auditory hallucinations are never seen except in a potential schizophrenic. The familiar aspects of schizophrenic thinking — condensation, omissions, neologisms or psychotic thought processes — are absent under LSD. There is a consistent harmony between thought and mood content under LSD which never produces a delusional process.

The drug has in latter years assumed a considerable importance in the treatment of psychoneurosis, but a study of the literature indicates that there is considerable disagreement regarding the types of patients for which the drug is beneficial and how it works. Some authorities are of the opinion that it is of the greatest value in the obsessional and anxiety groups, accompanied by mental tension (Sandison *et al.*, 1954; Cutner, 1959). Others quoted by Cohen (1960) exclude obsessional, compulsive, hysterical or acutely anxious or agitated patients. Some consider that the best results are obtained with psychopathic personalities and the worst with chronic tension states (Martin, 1957). All who have used this drug claim that it is a valuable aid to psychotherapy and regard the drug as a "deep" abreactive agent in that in certain cases it erupts early traumatic experiences as far back as infancy with appropriate emotional catharsis, which is believed to be of considerable therapeutic benefit to the patient. Attention has been drawn to the fact that the responses are not always indicative of the therapeutic value of the drug and indeed these vary enormously in some patients. Other patients who have a very severe reaction seem not to benefit, while others again in whom there is apparently no abreactive response get better.

There is some divergence of opinion as to how the drug produces its therapeutic effects. Some authorities stress the value of the abreactive qualities of the drug with the need for the re-integration of emerging unconscious material, but others stress the value of childhood experiences, whereas others again (Sandison, 1954) lay emphasis on archetypal sym-

References p. 221

bolic experiences. The effect of the LSD experience on the transference situation and the role played by the therapist have been regarded as highly significant.

The results claimed in the treatment of neurosis and personality disorders appear to be much influenced by the personality, aims and expectations of the therapist and the setting in which the drug is administered.

In spite of the considerable literature available, there has only recently been evidence of any controlled assessment of LSD-25 compared with other therapies. An attempt has been made to fill this gap by work at Roffey Park where Robinson and his colleagues have carried out a controlled assessment of the value of LSD-25 with Standard Therapy and combined hexobarbitone sodium (cyclonae and methedrine) in the treatment of 87 neurotic patients. Patients were assessed at the end of treatment and follow-up studies made 3 months and 6 months after discharge. Their investigations were carried out in a hospital environment designed for the short-term inpatients. At this hospital the patients were fully mobile and so could take part in all the activities of the hospital, such as occupational therapy, competitive games, dances, discussions, so that strong feelings of fellowship and mutual help were engendered. Psycholytic drugs were merely given as part of a comprehensive regime which fosters strong feelings of fellowship and mutual support amongst patients, and encourages a positive responsible attitude in human relations (Robinson et al., 1962).

Within this environment three groups of patients randomly selected were treated respectively with Standard Therapy, LSD-25 and a combination of cyclonal and methedrine. Irrespective of the method used, individual therapeutic sessions were held for each patient by the psychiatrist responsible for his treatment on an average of 3/4 hour three times weekly over a period of eight weeks.

By Standard Therapy these workers mean psychotherapy which may of course entail some abreaction either immediate or delayed. Such patients differed from the others only in that no drug was employed to produce an abreaction.

The design of the project based on random selection and allocation to each therapeutic group provided a controlled assessment of the value of each therapy in patients of similar social status, age groups, intelligence and sex distribution. All patients in the investigation were drawn mainly from Social Classes II and III, and about 70 per cent were classified as Superior or Bright Normal according to the Wechsler measurement of adult intelligence. The conclusions drawn from these investigations are as follows: the result of treatment showed no significant differences between the sexes nor in those married and single. Immediate results based on the clinical assessment of an independent outside consultant psychiatrist indicated that abreactive agents were less beneficial than Standard Therapy when used in the therapeutic community environment of the hospital. Standard Therapy and combined cyclonal and methedrine gave similar results in patients 3 months after discharge and both were better than results obtained with LSD-25. Six months after discharge the results obtained with Standard Therapy were better than those obtained with the abreactive agents used. However, results with LSD-25 were a little better than those obtained with cyclonal and methedrine. This controlled study indicates that abreactive therapy is less beneficial than Standard Therapy, and also shows that in general LSD-25 is superior to combined cyclonal and methedrine as an abreactive agent. It was somewhat gratifying to note that LSD-25 gave better immediate clinical results with patients whose symptoms were present for more than five years. This trend was not maintained, however, in follow-up studies and the conclusion reached is that, irrespective of treatment, the shorter the duration of symptoms the better the results. It would seem worth while doing further research into the value of LSD-25 in different personality structures. This study gives the impression that the passive dependent patient does significantly worse with LSD-25.

LSD was used in groups as an aid to group psychotherapy, but work on this is inconclusive. Further investigations in the use of this drug in both individual and group therapy are obviously necessary in order to determine the value and limitations of LSD as an aid to psychotherapy, but Robinson deserves some credit for carrying out the first controlled experiment in this field.

Sernyl (Phencyclidine)

Sernyl is 1-(1-phenylcyclohexyl)-piperidine. It was in fact first employed by anaesthetists because, when injected intravenously it caused a generalised insensitivity to pain without unconsciousness. Its clinical structure is closely similar to that of pethidine. This blocking of sensory impressions from the periphery occurs without any depression of heart or respiration. However the patients showed symptoms of a confused or schizoid character in the hours following, and its use as an anaesthetic was discontinued.

The drug acts selectively on the thalamus and midbrain and the EEG shows disappearance of alpha and beta rhythms and a definite slowing of the cortical rhythm especially in the occipital, temporal and parietal regions. Because of its probable effect on the thalamus, the drug was supposed to be an exteroceptive blocking agent, and its effects were likened to those of sensory deprivation. Davies and Beech (1960) gave the drug to patients who were then put into a sensory deprivation chamber and the subjects reported that their minds were being shut off from the outer world, as well as from visceroceptive stimuli ("sheer emptiness"). Most patients were inclined to vomit but the vomiting was not accompanied by nausea. This occurred even with low doses. After the session was over the patients reported that the experience had not been an unpleasant one. In fact the prevailing feeling is one of indifference. The commonest symptoms are that the patient cannot think clearly. It is "as if he had had a few drinks". He feels as if the doctor is a long distance away. He is tired, and he may want to fall asleep. There is often a constant humming sound in the head and this can be located as coming from the limbs, which feel heavy. They become insensitive to pinprick within the first half-hour, or hour. There is often a feeling that the hands or the arms are smaller or larger than normal. The patients have difficulty in answering questions of an abstract character, for instance about the meaning of proverbs. There is slight giddiness: after some 75 minutes the effects begin to wear off and after 2 hours the subject can walk about with perhaps only a faint feeling of giddiness. He may also feel that he is floating away or that people are in two dimensions, as if made of cardboard. There may occasionally be a fleeting state of catalepsy. Generally the subjects feel slowed up. On the whole the most important symptoms are depersonalisation, disturbances of time appreciation, euphoria, and restlessness, while the physical signs are dry mouth, vomiting, tremors, increased knee-jerks, and dilated pupils.

More troublesome symptoms are possible, such as negativism, agressiveness, or confusion.

One of Davies' patients was a serious obsessional individual and treatment with sernyl caused an increased memory for early experiences with repeated abreactions. Davies therefore tried out the drug on five different obsessionals with a total of some seventy treatments (Davies, 1960). His technique was to allow the patient to settle down in hospital. He took a full history and the patient had become accustomed to injections by receiving sodium amytal or methedrine on previous occasions. The patients were closely observed by the nursing staff and asked to write an account of the interview on the evening of the day on which it had occurred. The patient was given 5 to 10 mg of sernyl by mouth half an hour before the treatment was due. He had been given only a light meal previously.

The effects of the drug were to facilitate the flow of thought and to produce an abreaction in three cases out of five. Of five patients two were much improved, one was improved, and two were not improved. Davies emphasises that the treatment is only part of the total plan of therapy.

Conclusion

Luby and his colleagues (1959) as well as Davies and Beech (1960) have evaluated this drug, which is potent and relatively non-toxic. In some cases it makes the patient talkative and his memory of traumatic incidents in the past is enhanced. However it is doubtful if its effects are as satisfactory or free from danger as those of a combination or amylobarbitone and methedrine i.v., which are more commonly used.

Beech et al. (1961) are continuing their investigations of the alleged psychotogenic action of the drug. Up till now technical difficulties have prevented a full examination of the abnormal psychological effects.

Psilocybin

This drug is the active compound of an intoxicating mushroom which has been long used by Indians in Mexico for obtaining a euphoric and drunken state. It was identified only in 1958 and it was synthesised and given its present name (Hofmann, 1958).

References p. 221

Its effects have been found to be similar to those of LSD but the side-effects are less serious. A good account of it is given by Isbell (1959). The drug has an effect on the autonomic nervous system chiefly in the nature of a central sympathetic stimulation. The drug is chemically related to serotonin.

We have investigated the effects of psilocybin on a normal subject, a young male aged 25. He was given 6 mg by mouth. Subjective sensations were correlated with clinical symptoms and with the EEG, psycho-galvanic reflex, heart rate and respiration. The patient had previously been conditioned to react by fear to a particular tone.

The main findings were: *subjective sensations*. Euphoria, a feeling that everything was very comic, visual hallucinations of a multi-coloured cloud 2 feet above him, elongation and shrinking of the body, lack of insight. There was no hypermnesia for early or late events in his life, and he did not feel inclined to discuss his plans for the future.

Clinical symptoms: Mydriasis, greatest after two and a half hours, as also increase of the pulse rate from 70 to 120, hyperhidrosis, hypertonia of muscles and slight restlessness.

Polygraphic findings: Increased muscle potentials tended to interfere with EEG and cardiotachymetric records, but one and a half hours after the injection, the heart rate and the PGR failed to respond either to the conditional or unconditional stimulus although the respiration responded more markedly.

Conclusion: The drug has an action similar to that of LSD but the symptoms are not so marked. Side effects are less dangerous.

The effects of this drug were fully discussed at a symposium in 1961 in London.

CHAPTER 9

Anti-depressive Drugs

Amphetamine, Ritalin, Meratran, Preludin

Pharmacologically the amphetamines belong to the group of sympatho-mimetic amines, of which adrenaline and ephedrine are the standard representatives, although these last lack the pronounced stimulant effect on the cortex and the brain-stem. However the amphetamines have very little action on other bodily functions except in high doses. They are of exceptional interest and are used in a variety of conditions, but their effects are transitory and they treat symptoms rather than diseases. One of their uses is to counteract oversedation. They are also employed to produce abreaction, often when given at the same time as sodium amylo-barbitone. They are given to children, and even to children who are hyperactive and destructive. They will combat the withdrawal symptoms in morphine and other addictions, and they counteract fatigue. Some therapists unwisely prescribe them over a lengthy period to combat depression. Amphetamine is also used for Parkinsonism, and for narco-lepsy, when combined with atropine. Another common use is to counter excessive appetite in obese patients. As well as amphetamine, there is dextro-amphetamine (dexedrine) and methamphetamine (methedrine).

Methamphetamine is the most potent of the three, and 5 mg correspond to 8 mg or 9 mg of amphetamine. Dexedrine has a greater ratio of adrenergic effects on the brain and produces fewer autonomic side-effects. However individuals react differently to these three drugs and one cannot tell in advance to which they will react most favourably. Their extracerebral effects are mostly in raising the blood pressure and in constricting peripheral blood vessels. They relax the bronchial muscles, thereby easing asthma and they diminish peristalsis and they dilate the pupils. However these effects are relatively unimportant compared with the central euphoriant effect (Swanson and Smith, 1961).

References p. 221

We have found that one of the best agents for abreaction is to give some 5 mg to 10 mg of methedrine i.v., combined with about 200 mg of sodium amylobarbitone. The effect of this combination varies from patient to patient. The most common effect is for the patient to have a feeling of well-being and relaxation and to have an urge to talk indefinitely about his psychological conflicts. Patients are suggestible under the treatment and this fact can be utilised by the therapist. This treatment has one benefit which has not so far been described to our knowledge. This is in the case of some agitated depressions. The patient may have been ill for a very long time and have lost all hope, but when he has an intravenous injection of these two drugs he has a feeling of excessive well-being and calm and finds that he can write letters and do things which he has not been able to do for perhaps years. This gives him a picture of what he might be like when he recovers, and the experience offers him a new hope which enables him to co-operate much more with the psychiatrist. A few tense patients however have said that they feel "jittery" when under the influence of amphetamine, and they have a "hang-over" the next day. However in such patients the giving of perphenazine has a similar effect in giving the patient renewed energy but accompanied by a feeling of calm, and their work proceeds in a more orderly and steady manner, and there is no "hang-over".

Rather surprisingly some paediatricians give very large doses of amphetamine to children over a long period in the treatment of enuresis. The rationale of this is that such children sleep very deeply and so lose control of their sphincters during the night, and the amphetamine is supposed to make them sleep more lightly. We have however found ill effects from this treatment on the children and we have preferred to use hypnosis and suggestion in such cases. Such patients can be trained both to use their bladders as reservoirs to a greater extent by day and also to sleep more lightly at night.

There is a strong feeling on the Continent that general practitioners should not use tranquillising drugs but they should send such patients to psychiatrists to supervise their treatment. This is particularly true of cases of depression, as practitioners too often prescribe amphetamine and the less effective MAOI's and imipramine without having much notion of the indications or the dosage range of these drugs or their side-effects. One has found patients being treated with amphetamine, or with amphetamine combined with barbiturates over very long periods of time so that the patients became addicts. Amphetamine is a drug of addiction and it is not unusual for some patients to increase their dosage to as much as 75 mg a day. Many cases of shop-lifting among women have occurred in those who take amphetamine. Murders may also be committed by amphetamine addicts. Up till recently it has been a habit among certain youths to boil up pieces of paper soaked in amphetamine and in this way they can take as much as 250 mg in a day. Such youths may go almost without food or sleep for a fortnight. I have seen two such youths who had committed murder when under the influence of amphetamine. Incidentally in both cases there were schizophrenic symptoms as described in amphetamine addiction by Connell (1958). Patients describe to us vividly how under the influence of amphetamine they give way to impulses to rape, steal or murder. The drug can inhibit any ability to feel compassion or to visualise the results of their crimes.

In our experience the use of amphetamine has led to addiction to alcohol or other drugs at a later date.

Another youth who had a criminal record and who was an addict stated that his arms and legs were quite insensitive when under the influence of amphetamine. This is a characteristic of intoxication with sernyl which has a similar chemical structure to that of amphetamine.

Connell has described schizophreniform psychoses with clear intellect in patients who are addicts to amphetamine but in these patients the psychosis is terminated by withdrawal of the drug.

Methylphenidate hydrochloride (ritalin) produces psychic effects similar to, but relatively weaker than the amphetamines, while apparently lacking many of the autonomic side-effects of the latter. It has been used in conjunction with reserpine to counteract its depressant effect.

Pipradol hydrochloride (meratran) produces a stimulant effect somewhat similar to the amphetamines but with less euphoria, less anorexia and with rather less insomnia than the latter. The effects however do not appear to be uniformly reliable if one may judge from reports on the drug which have appeared up till now.

Preludin (phenmetrazine) was developed in Germany. It is rather less euphoriant than amphetamine and is used in 25 mg tablets *t.d.s.* half an hour before meals for obesity. It had led to severe addiction in some cases.

To conclude, one may say that amphetamine is a useful drug as an occasional stimulant and to counteract a transitory depression. It should never be given for more than one course of treatment, such as for obesity, and not for more than three months. Nowadays, there are non-euphoriant drugs such as lucofen* (Warner) which counteract appetite. These are preferable to the amphetamines. In psychiatry it is probably used most widely to produce an abreaction. Some believe that abreactions caused by methedrine or amytal are just as effective as those obtained by the use of LSD or psilocybin. We would be inclined to agree with this but there are a number of psychiatrists with wide experience in the use of the so-called psycholytic drugs who ar most enthusiastic over their results with these more powerful agents.

Imipramine (tofranil)

The anti-depressive properties of this drug were discovered by Kuhn in 1957 in Switzerland. Owing to its chemical structure, which resembles that of the phenothiazines, it was at first used for schizophrenia, but Kuhn soon discovered that it had a marked anti-depressive action. The S atom is absent in the centre ring which is 7-sided but the same side-chain is attached to the N atom (see appendix).

Pharmacological properties

Like chlorpromazine it depresses the reticular formation. It blocks the effect of a pain stimulus so that it does not cause an alerting reaction in a dozing animal, as shown in the EEG. It also activates the rhinencephalon like chlorpromazine and in high doses can produce convulsions.

Some of its pharmacological actions constitute the side-effects of the drug. Most of these consist of atropine-like effects. There is a dry mouth which however is not very disagreeable. Marked sweating can be more of a problem. The sweat has a characteristic chemical odour which clings even to the patient's bed. There is sometimes difficulty in accommodating because of mydriasis. With higher doses there may be urinary retention. Constipation which is common in depression becomes more marked. Postural hypotension can occur with consequent vertigo. Partly because of this, falls in elderly patients can constitute a serious danger. The

---

* Approved name chlorphentermine.

hypotension has been considered responsible for some cardiac accidents. In elderly people a close watch should be kept on the heart and blood pressure. Tachycardia may be as high as 130. Sometimes there is a fine tremor and this occurs in some 10 per cent of cases but especially with high doses in elderly patients. Insomnia is also common. At any stage there may be a switch-over to a hypomanic reaction (English, 1961).

Kuhn (1960) has pointed out that clinically there are two responses in patients, either a sympathotonic reaction in which there is restlessness, insomnia and agitation, or else there is a vagotonic effect characterised by tiredness and somnolence. He therefore recommends that at the beginning of treatment 25 mg be given to a patient at bedtime. If the drug accentuates the tendency to sleep, then it can be given throughout the day with confidence. If however the effect is one of insomnia and restlessness, then it should not be administered after 3.00 *p.m.* Agranulocytosis can occur (Bird, 1960).

Dosage

The usual dosage is one 25 mg tablet three times a day, and one gradually increases the dose by one tablet every day until the patient is having eight in the day. This is continued until the symptoms remit, and after that dosage is reduced to a maintenance level. This however may require to be as high as 200 mg daily, but may be much less. Old people are more susceptible to drugs in general and because of the danger of falls, smaller tablets of 10 mg are supplied.

A special course of treatment of an intensive character which begins with injections of 25 mg i.m. and ends with oral administration is recommended on the basis of Kuhn's work. The drug is probably destroyed to some extent in the stomach so that the i.m. route is more effective and the beneficial results come on more quickly than in the usual 3 or 4 days.

Side-effects

Some of these have been mentioned above. In addition there may be itching of the skin and loss of appetite and there may be some confusion, with visual hallucinations. In such cases treatment should be stopped and a phenothiazine substituted. It is inadvisable to stop the treatment

References p. 221

suddenly, as the depression may be increased or the patient may suffer from extreme lethargy. Parkinsonian symptoms have been reported!

On the whole however serious side-effects occur only with doses of 300 mg a day or more, or else in patients who are elderly or who have suffered from renal or other diseases.

The drug should not be given together with MAOI's; they are incompatible and can cause confusion. Also it should not be given within a week of the patient having had a MAOI. It should be given with caution in cases of agitation, but it combines well with librium for such patients. The librium can be given in doses of 30 to 40 mg a day.

Results of treatment

It is generally agreed that imipramine is the drug which has been established as the most effective against depression. This applies particularly to the psychotic type. Some reports describe some 30 per cent recoveries and another 30 per cent who are greatly improved. Unlike the MAOI's tofranil does not help cases of anxiety nor the atypical neurotic depressions. It does not help retarded schizophrenics though they may show more activity for a time. Usually their hallucinations and delusions are enhanced. There have been numerous controlled clinical trials. Lehmann et al. (1958) showed that the drug was definitely superior to a placebo while Ball and Kiloh (1959) obtained a recovery rate of 74 per cent in endogenous depressions and 59 per cent in reactive depressions, compared with 22 per cent and 20 per cent respectively for the placebo. These controlled studies as well as others (Holt et al., 1960; Miller et al., 1960; Sloane et al., 1959) support uncontrolled studies such as those of Blair (1960) who found that imipramine could be successful in cases of chronic depression where all previous therapy had failed. It often succeeded in patients where ECT could not be carried out, whether because of serious illness, refusal of the treatment by the patient or because of difficult veins. Blair quotes figures which are more favourable than those quoted by most other authors. In a series of 100 patients, 59 per cent made a full recovery while 20 per cent in addition were much improved. Fleminger and Groden (1962) had 55 per cent good results (see also Part I, Chapter 7).

Imipramine in comparison with ECT

It is difficult to asses the relative value of two treatments in a disease which is itself likely to clear up spontaneously. This is particularly so if the advocates of a drug state that it must be continued for several months before there is to be an admission of failure. Bruce *et al.* (1960) assigned patients in a random manner to ECT and tofranil. The number treated was 50. Their conclusion was that the proportion of patients who improved during the first month of treatment was higher in the group given ECT but over 60 per cent of those given tofranil showed a good response in that time, perhaps justifying the view that tofranil may often serve as a substitute for ECT.

One advantage of ECT is that one can predict that if one gives 8 ECT's there is likely to be an immediate response. On the other hand it is likely that one would require to go on giving maintenance doses of tofranil until the illness has come to a spontaneous conclusion. There is sometimes a necessity for urgent action not only where there is a danger of suicide but also of severe inanition. One cannot tell beforehand if a patient will respond better to one or other treatment but there is a consensus of opinion that both treatments act on the same kind of patient. Sometimes a patient however responds to ECT after failing with imipramine and vice versa. The two treatments go quite well together. Concentrated ECT however is more effective for agitated melancholia than imipramine.

Carstairs (1961) suggests that perhaps imipramine and other drugs may be more effective than ECT in preventing a second attack, but in our experience ECT is more effective in this respect. This is especially so if it is used just before the next attack is expected in recurrent cases.

Arnold *et al.* (1960) recommend giving 4 ECT's prior to imipramine, claiming that secondary effects are diminished. We often give 150 to 200 mg of tofranil daily after the eight ECT's. If the patient is agitated, 20 or 30 mg of librium daily may be added during the ECT course. After the symptoms have abated we continue with 150 mg of tofranil daily. Again if restlessness is combined with the depression, librium which has a slightly sedative effect should also be added in doses of 20 to 30 mg daily.

We still believe that on the whole, too little rather than too much ECT is given in the depression. At one hospital where ECT's are discon-

References p. 221

tinued as soon as the depression remits, two-thirds of the patients relapse within a few weeks. Relapses do not occur to the same extent if a minimum course of 8 treatments is given.

A recent account by Kiloh and Ball (1961) of imipramine in relation to ECT is of interest. These writers describe a six-month follow-up of 97 patients treated with imipramine. Maximal improvement could occur between 1½ and 4 weeks after the start of the treatment. They suggest however that ECT be used if the maximal effect is slow in appearing. They found that in endogenous depression 55 cases (66 per cent) showed an initial response. There was however an 18 per cent relapse in 6 months, half of the relapsed cases having ceased to take the drug because of side-effects. Kemp *et al.* (1961) had similar results.

Imipramine in comparison with MAOI's

Most writers have found that imipramine is superior to the MAOI's in the treatment of psychotic depressions. Controlled trials have supported this opinion. Miller *et al.* (1960) in treating chronic depressions where the prognosis was not so good as usual found that 30 per cent gave a satisfactory response to imipramine therapy but rather less satisfactory results were obtained with iproniazid, amphetamine and a placebo. Holt *et al.* (1960) found that phenelzine gave the best results and then marplan, and imipramine came only third in relieving symptoms of depression. This view however is a minority one.

As will be seen later phenelzine (nardil) and possibly other MAOI's are more successful in dealing with atypical depressions where there are some neurotic or hysterical symptoms superadded (Sargant, 1961).

Conclusion

Imipramine is a valuable addition to our methods of treating endogenous depression. It does not merely remove symptoms as amphetamine does, but after a course of treatment the patient feels well. After the initial improvement or recovery the dose can be reduced to the maintenance level. The treatment is a useful adjuvant to ECT, but where the latter is contra-indicated, an equally good result may often be obtained. On the other hand in the case of a reactive or neurotic depression phenelzine is preferable in the opinion of many writers, especially if combined with librium. It is useful also in enuresis (Munster *et al.*, 1961).

Amitriptyline

This drug was developed originally in Denmark and there was a symposium on the drug in America in 1961.

The chemical structure is similar to that of imipramine but there is a substitution of C for N where the promazine side-chain is attached.

This change causes a more sedative action while retaining the anti-depressive quality of the drug. It also has neuroleptic qualities similar to those of chlorprothixene (taractan), which also has this C-formation as well as the same side-chain. Neither drug ordinarily causes Parkinsonian side-effects despite the neuroleptic action (see appendix).

Pharmacology

In experimental animals the drug causes sedation, and inhibition of spontaneous activity. In small doses it abolishes conditioned reactions without affecting the unconditioned responses, thus resembling chlor-promazine. As with barbiturates however both responses are abolished in higher dosage. Like imipramine it potentiates anaesthetics and also has a hypotensive action. It increases the heart rate. Its action is similar to that of chlorpromazine in counteracting the effects of adrenaline. It is a strong anti-histaminic.

Its toxicity to mice is slightly less than that of imipramine.

Dosage

The usual dosage for adults is 50 mg orally *t.d.s.* but the dose can be gradually increased by 25 mg a day. Usually it is not necessary to exceed 200 to 250 mg a day but up to 450 mg daily has been given.

It can be administrated i.m. or slowly i.v. in doses of 50 mg. For geriatric patients, tablets are of 10 mg as with imipramine. If a quick result is desired the patient may be given 50 to 100 mg daily i.m. A changeover to oral therapy is made after 2 days or so.

For many patients 150 mg daily is adequate. Improvement occurs within 1 or 2 weeks. Otherwise the dose is gradually raised to 300 mg daily. Side-effects however are likely to be troublesome at doses over 200 mg daily. As soon as the depression comes under control, the dose is reduced to the maintenance level which is usually 150 mg daily.

Side-effects and dangers

It should be remembered that the drug potentiates sedatives such as barbiturates, anaesthetics and alcohol. It it incompatible with MAOI's. In depressed patients there is an ever-present danger of suicide. It should not be given to patients with glaucoma or with difficulties of micturition.

These side-effects are the same as for imipramine except that the tendency to insomnia and anxiety is less (Pressman and Weiss, 1961).

Clinical effects

Feldman (1961) thought that the drug was at least as effective as imipramine and slightly superior to nialamide. He considered that it was definitely superior to nardil and librium for depression. The target symptoms affected were tension in 67 per cent of cases, lack of energy in 62 per cent, loss of appetite in 58 per cent, lack of interest in the environment in 56 per cent and loss of sleep 51 per cent.

Dorfman (1961) found that side-effects such as dry mouth and sweating began to show with doses of 225 mg daily. He found that it was useful in anxiously depressed patients. Ayd (1961 a) used it for involutional, cyclic, neurotic, and schizoid depressions but added amphetamines, barbiturates or phenothiazines where necessary. Of 130 patients, 31 per cent showed marked improvement and another 48 per cent some improvement. The beneficial effects came on quicker and were apparent with comparatively low doses (75 to 100 mg daily). Mild psychotic patients responded best. Oltman and Friedman (1961 b) claim it to be equal to tofranil but with fewer side-effects.

Conclusion

The action of this drug is similar to those of imipramine but it is claimed that the effects come on more quickly and that the side-effects, particularly those of anxiety and insomnia are less marked. There is also claimed to be a slightly neuroleptic effects similar to that of chlorprothixen (taractan).

In our experience the effect of ECT are generally much better than those produced by this class of drug. However it may be a useful adjuvant to ECT. Both forms of treatment are used for the same type of case. Where ECT is contra-indicated this drug may be successful. At the present time however the value of imipramine as a successful anti-depressant has been more firmly established.

Monoamine oxidase inhibitors

This class includes the following drugs: iproniazid (marsilid), isocarboxazid (marplan), nialamide (niamid), tranylcypromine (parnate) and phenelzine (nardil). The other two classes of anti-depressant drugs are those of the amphetamine group, and thirdly imipramine and amitriptyline.

A good account of these drugs is given by Vernier (1961). Our appendix at the end shows the principal members of the group, while it gives as well the major pharmacological actions of these drugs. All are hydrazines except tranylcypromine known commercially as parnate. A hydrazine compound has the following structure, $R_1 - NH - NH - R_2$.

It will be noticed that tranylcypromine contains a phenylethylamine nucleus which relates them to the amphetamine group.

Their effects on behaviour however are different from those caused by amphetamine. In animals amphetamine causes over-activity immediately after injection, while MAOI's often cause depression of activity initially. However the laboratory test which appears to provide an analogue of their clinical anti-depressant action is that where chronic treatment with iproniazid in the case of rats maintains their activity of running in exercise wheels at much higher levels than controls. Numerous laboratories have supported the original observation that brain serotonin concentration rises after the administration of MAOI's. The significance of this however with regard to their clinical effect in removing depression still remains unclear.

Whereas imipramine in large doses can cause convulsions, the action of MAOI's is to raise the threshold for electrically induced convulsions.

References p. 221

Pre-treatment with MAOI's inhibits the sedative action of reserpine as well as its mentally depressing effect.

MAOI's have a potentiating effect on certain drugs including anaesthetics and are contra-indicated with phenothiazines (Casey *et al.,* 1961).

These drugs also have a partially paralysing effect on smooth muscles which accounts for the production of constipation and dysuria as well as the lowering of blood pressure. It is thus also responsible for orthostatic hypotension. Some workers have described an analgesic action of iproniazid which might explain its success in cases of angina.

In animals toxic actions have been noted on the liver and on the blood. The drugs also tend to raise the body temperature.

The use of MAOI's in depressive states

The use of these drugs began as early as 1951 in America when it was noticed that tuberculous patients treated with iproniazid showed improved appetite and more energy and a greater feeling of well-being. However it was not until 1957 that a special Congress met to discuss their usefulness and thereafter a great deal of clinical and biochemical research ensued (Loomer *et al.,* 1957).

Estimation of the effects of drugs on psychotic and atypical depressions

There are some difficulties in estimating the effect of drugs on this type of illness. Depression is often a self-limiting illness. For this reason it is difficult to be sure that the remission has occurred as the result of a given drug. This is particularly so when the advocates of a drug insist that it may take three weeks or more to take effect and that is must be kept up for a period of some three months. This is in marked contrast to the effects of ECT where the favourable effect may be expected after some four treatments. Some advocates of this type of drug have recently shifted their ground. It has been generally agreed that imipramine and now amitriptyline are more successful in the treatment of psychotic depressions and the MAOI's have been advocated to a greater extent for the so-called typical neurotic or hysterical depressions. Here again there is difficulty in estimating the effects of the drug. The MAOI is often given in conjunction with another drug, generally librium, and so it is difficult to estimate which drug is the more important in bringing about an improvement.

It is just in this class of case where social and psychological factors are more likely to be significant. It is difficult to eliminate entirely the placebo effect or the milieu effect.

Despite all this, the general consensus of opinion is that there is a definite place in psychiatry for the use of these drugs (Bates and Douglas, 1961).

Plan of treatment

Most of these agents take an average of three weeks to show their effect although parnate may be expected to act more quickly. They must be continued until a spontaneous remission occurs. However it is advisable to reduce the dose to the lowest possible level after the desired effect has been achieved.

Kline (1961) however takes the view that too many physicians give too low a dose, particularly at the beginning of treatment. He maintains that the dosage required bears no relation to the severity of the symptoms. It is an all-or-nothing reaction. If side-effects occur, he does not at once lower the dose but tries as a rule to treat the side-effects. He claims that many patients come to him who are receiving the correct drugs but in sub-threshold dosage. When this is corrected, beneficial effects eventually are noted.

This point of view is controversial and has perhaps led to the dosage of psychotropic drugs being higher in America than elsewhere. Kline prefers to use drugs rather than ECT, limiting the use of the latter to cases of potential suicide.

MAOI's in psychotic depression

The work of Sargant and his co-workers and also of Rees and Davies (1961) in England among others have demonstrated that these are potent and effective drugs and that their success cannot be explained merely by placebo effects or as the result of the additional care and supervision given to the patient. However almost no clinicians have claimed that the

References p. 221

effects of these drugs are superior to those of ECT.

Notes on individual members of this group

(1) Marsilid: This compound has been considered by some to be the most effective clinically of this group. However the absence of a satisfactory test for liver function which would enable the clinician to recognise which patients are susceptible to liver damage has militated against its suitability for use in psychiatry. The drug has been withdrawn from the market in certain parts of the world as also has pheniprazine (cavodil, catron).

In England marplan has been used insead of marsilid because it was believed also to be less toxic. It was claimed that it is very much more effective as a MAOI but in the opinion of Sargant (1961) it is only a little less effective than marsilid (Joshi, 1961).

Even the successors of marsilid are not free from danger, for fatal cardiovascular changes have been reported with a patient on nardil. King (1959) and Paredes *et al.* (1961) have reported a similar experience with marplan. Up to date however no such side-effects have been reported with nialamide (niamid), but niamid is generally considered to have a less potent therapeutic effect.

It is agreed that marplan is less toxic than the two drugs which have been withdrawn but it is more potent than niamid (Freeman *et al.*, 1960).

King (1959) believes that psychotic patients do better with ECT than they do with phenelzine. He had one fatal case from cardiovascular changes with the drug.

(2) Phenelzine: This drug differs from marplan in its pharmacological effect. From the chemical standpoint it resembles amphetamine to some extent but is also a MAOI. It is more likely to develop states of excitation and hypomanic episodes than some of the other MAOI inhibitors (Imlah, 1960). There were two controlled studies in England (Harris *et al.*, 1960 and Middlefell *et al.*, 1960). The former found that there was no advantage of phenelzine over a placebo for psychotic depressions but the second study found that the drug was more potent than a placebo. Hutchinson and Smedberg (1960) in a controlled trial obtained 64 per cent good results in depression (see also appendix).

(3) Tranylcypromine (parnate): This is a MAOI which is not a hydrazine and it is structurally related to the amphetamine-like phenelzine. Its effects come on much more quickly and its action does not last so long as the other MAOI's after its withdrawal. For this reason the danger of suicide at the beginning of treatment is lessened. It is given in doses of 5 to 20 mg daily. The effects may come on within 24 hours. The side-effects include insomnia, and mild hypotension. If the patients suffer from anxiety this symptom is likely to be accentuated and for this reason it is combined by the makers with stelazine. This effect of promoting psychomotor activity and wakefulness is probably related to its structural similarity to amphetamine (see also Lesse, 1961; Lurie and Salzer, 1961).

Another MAOI called etryptamine (monase) was put on the market but has since been withdrawn. It did not appear to have any advantages over other MAOI's. It was recommended for use in conjunction with other measures for depression but was too toxic.

MAOI's in the treatment of atypical depression

Berger (1960) has written as follows: "In therapeutic application, tranquillisers and anti-depressants may differ from each other much less than is generally assumed. Certain tranquilizers such as meprobamate alone or in combination with benactyzine have been reported to be of value in the treatment of all types of depression".

We have also noted that piperazines such as perphenazine have energizing and euphoriant effects. Recently Sargant and Dally (1962) have suggested that MAOI's might be of use in treating cases of atypical depression. In a group of 60 patients, they reported that there was no clear demarcation between typical depressions and anxiety states. Many anxiety states were found to respond equally well to treatment with MAOI's preferably when in combination with librium. Their 60 patients had been diagnosed as cases of atypical depression, anxiety hysteria, or anxiety neurosis. Fifteen patients responded to a MAOI alone, 28 did best with a MAOI combined with librium and 17 failed to respond to a MAOI but they responded to librium. They still used iproniazid in some cases but this was exceptional "owing to its somewhat toxic effects on the liver."

With regard to this paper one may remark that when MAOI's are given, the anxiety symptoms disappear before the symptoms of depression. The drug often took 4 to 8 days to take effect and it was not expected that the maximal effect against depression would be reached for 10 days. They take care to see that fainting and giddiness do not mask the beneficial effects. They remark that occasional cases of jaundice are starting to be reported with nearly all the MAOI's as well as with iproniazid. Another recent study was that of Hare *et al.* (1962) who carried out a double blind investigation. In it they compared phenelzine both with dexamphetamine and with a placebo. The test however lasted for only 10 days. They found that anxiety, but not depression, was relieved in a significant number of their cases and they suggested that the benefits of phenelzine in depressive states might simply be due to a sedative action and that it might have no anti-depressant effect at all. It would appear that this was true as far as their study went, but this lasted only 10 days and it is known that the MAOI's affect anxiety before they influence depression. It is well established that MAOI's do affect depression and that there is often even a swing-over to the manic phase. It must be remembered that there is a high degree of spontaneous recovery in depressive states.

In cases of atypical and neurotic depression, as here, the actual effect of drugs is often not so important as psychotherapy. Drugs can never constitute the whole treatment of anxiety.

Side-effects and dangers of MAOI drugs

It is essential for the clinician to realise that under certain circumstances these drugs are dangerous. He should also know what side-effects can appear. The following are some of the more important (Ayd, 1961 a and b).

(1) Potentiation of a drug: The clinician may notice that a patient is excessively drowsy or again that he is excessively active. These symptoms may be caused by the fact that the patient is also taking either a barbiturate or excessive quantities of coffee and these drugs are being potentiated by the MAOI's. Sometimes a doctor gives amphetamine at the beginning before the MAOI has time to take effect. There then comes a time when the MAOI potentiates the amphetamine.

(2) Liver toxicity: This has already been mentioned in the case of marsilid and cavodil. It also constitutes a danger for marplan. As soon as jaundice appears the drug should be withdrawn. Since the drugs are not essential for the treatment of depression it is difficult to justify the giving of a drug which may cause the death of a patient by necrosis of the liver.

(3) Hypotension: This effect can be avoided if the patient does not bend down but rather squats. It is also necessary to give the patient a full diet, and a food such as complan may be added to his usual diet. Great care should be given in treating a patient with cardiovascular disease because of the deaths reported.

(4) Neuralgia: It is thought that the drugs diminish the patient's ability to utilise the Vitamin B complex and in consequence twitchings of muscles and vague neuralgic pains may result. These should be treated by Vitamin B preparations.

(5) Constipation: This again is caused by the partially paralysing effect on smooth muscle which causes the fall in blood pressure.

(6) Dysuria: This can occur, and the drug should not be given to cases with prostatic illness.

(7) Reduced sexual capacity: The reflexes are slower and for this reason the drugs have been used for the treatment of ejaculatio praecox.

(8) Oedema: This can occur, and occasionally a diuretic is necessary.
   Other disagreeable symptoms are sweating, blurred vision, dry mouth, potentiation of schizophrenic symptoms and agranulocytosis.

Conclusion

In 1957 when the MAOI's were launched in a big way for the benefit of psychiatrists it appeared that they were safe and that the biochemists were on the point of presenting a clear pathology of one of the important psychoses, namely melancholia. It was thought that mental depression was caused by a lack of serotonin and other amines in the brain and that these drugs would raise the level of this substance and so cause the melancholia to remit. These hopes however have not been fulfilled but nevertheless interest in these drugs has led to many important discoveries in the biochemical field.

The second disappointment has been the toxicity of some of these drugs. The chief deleterious action has been on the liver but deaths have also occurred from their effect on the heart.

Their delayed action has also been a disadvantage, as well as their continued action after being withdrawn. Most writers have reported that imipramine and amitriptyline are definitely superior, and this has lessened the importance of this class of agent.

Another fact which has lessened their importance is the superiority of ECT if it is given with the correct technique.

However most psychiatrists will agree with Sargant that there is a class of patient who appears to be chronically depressed or anxious or a combination of the two but in whose case there does not appear to be sufficient environmental cause for their psychological state. In these instances the effect of such drugs as librium are definitely enhanced if a MAOI such as phenelzine is given in addition. If these drugs are given for a time, an opportunity is provided for enabling the patients to readjust their lives and also break the habit of having an anxious and depressed outlook.

There have been some attacks on the MAOI's, particularly the hydrazines. Ayd (1961 a) for instance concludes that "the future of the hydrazine MAOI's is dim indeed. Unless there is an improvement in this type of medicine, they will become obsolete because of their limited usefulness and the hazards of their prolonged administration. Thus they will be driven from the market and join marsilid and catron on the shelf of discarded pharmaceuticals. At the moment and for the immediate future it appears to be more advantageous and safer to treat melancholic individuals with amitriptyline and imipramine."

Again, Wilcox (1961) finds he can treat psychiatric out-patients successfully although employing psychotropic drugs only to a minimal extent. He prefers to leave his patients in an alert state. He says "I am appalled when I read and hear about the complex and hidden side-effects that accompany the use of so many of the new drugs widely heralded in psychopharmocology." He believes that methods of psychotherapy and one or other technique of electrocerebral treatment should be used in the first place. He thinks that psychotropic drugs should only be given to patients in hospital when other measures have failed. It has been found that when this policy is employed remarkably few patients require to go to hospital.

In our experience many patients are unwilling to continue taking pills week after week without being convinced that they still require them.

It is possible that in the future electrocerebral treatment will be more studied and used. We still prefer to employ it in cases of severe chronic neurosis. This often breaks the habit of depression and anxiety and a number of patients have written to us later to say that the effects of treatment have been lasting, despite the previous chronicity of the condition.

General principles in the treatment of depression

(1) The amphetamine group of drugs can be used to relieve symptoms but should not be given after 3.00 *p.m.* and a barbiturate hypnotic should be given at night. It is often advisable to combine the amphetamine with a mild dose of barbiturate given at the same time in the proportion of 5 mg of amphetamine to 100 mg of amylobarbitone. Amphetamine however should be given only for symptomatic relief for short periods until spontaneous recovery occurs. Amphetamines produce tolerance so that courses should not exceed three weeks. A proportion of patients are apt to commit anti-social acts with a dosage of 10 mg or more.

(2) Atypical depression may have been precipitated by environmental stress so that psychotherapy and rehabilitation may be the main plank in treatment. Endogenous and reactive factors vary in relative importance, but the resulting symptomatology may be the same. Physical health also influences mood so that diet and exercise can be a useful adjunct to treatment.

(3) Chronic and severe depression may not respond to ECT at a given point of time but may do so at a later date.

(4) Of the anti-depressive drugs which act indirectly, imipramine and possibly amitriptyline are the best. Their greatest success is in cases of psychotic depression and they are used if ECT is contra-indicated or if its

effects are unsatisfactory. They can be given coincidentally and follow-ing ECT.

(5) Imipramine and the MAOI's must be kept at a maintenance dose until it is evident or likely that spontaneous recovery has set in.

(6) As patients are unwilling in many cases to take pills indefinitely and as the MAOI's produce side-effects before they produce therapeutic effects, the patient is likely to refuse to continue this type of treatment. It is better therefore to explain this to the patient and to a responsible relative to ensure that a full course is given.

Some of these comments are based on a presentation of the views of the late A. Kennedy by D. Leigh (Kennedy, 1961).

CHAPTER 10

The Treatment of Alcoholism

There has been a marked change in the prognosis of alcoholism during the past 10 years. This has partly been due to a better understanding of its pathology and partly to a change of attitude on the part of the public to the alcoholic patient. The greatest single factor in helping the alcoholic has been the world-wide movement known as "Alcoholics Anonymous". This is an association of individuals who have recognised that alcohol is a problem for them and that therefore they cannot drink. They make it possible for a patient, preferably after medical treatment, to join their circle and learn how to live as a non-drinker in a drinker's world*.

When a chronic alcoholic is brought for treatment to a medical man during an acute exacerbation of symptoms, the first indications are to put him to bed, detoxicate him, chiefly by injection intravenously of fluids containing glucose and vitamins, and to sedate him and provide simple nourishment. Treatment will be necessary for his gastritis and he should be guarded against respiratory infection.

In the past, opinions have been divided as to whether the sudden withdrawal of alcohol facilitates the onset of delirium tremens. If the patient is very ill, it is arguable that he should continue for a time with alcohol as it provides him with calories and keeps him sedated to a certain extent. The difficulty that alcohol by mouth is likely to enhance the gastritis can be obviated by giving some preparation like "Curethyl" (Bengue) intravenously. This contains alcohol as well as vitamin B and glucose.

The common practice however is to give very high doses of vitamins B and C, intravenously. "Parentrovite", provided in ampoules of 10 ml, contains very high concentrations of aneurine, riboflavine, pyridoxine, nicotinamide and ascorbic acid, together with dextrose. As much as 20 ml

---

* Some psychiatrists believe wrongly that it is not worthwhile sending non-religious patients to AA. This is an error. Some members are agnostics, who say that they like to live "in tune with nature", rather than "in accordance with Gods will"!

can be given at a time. Sometimes there is a sudden and dramatic disappearance of the symptoms of terror and agitation during the giving of the injection. It is important however that such injections should not be given if there is any hint of heart failure and decompensation.

The most commonly used sedatives are amylobarbitone or sodium amylobarbitone in doses of 9 to 18 grains (600 to 1,200 mg) daily. Librium in doses of 10 to 20 mg *t.d.s.* can also be given. For more severe excitements an i.m. injection of chlorpromazine 50 mg may be given.

Nourishment

It is not always realised that the appetite of an alcoholic can only be stimulated by tasty and savoury foods. He is most likely to accept beef tea with an egg in it and fingers of toast, or again, if he is less ill, a plate of cold ham, calf's foot jelly or chicken. Concentrated food powders such as complan which contain the necessary calories, vitamins, minerals and salts should be given if possible.

Psychological considerations

The important points to get across to the patient are as follows:

(1) that although he is seriously ill, there is a cure for his illness.

(2) that there has been a change of attitude towards alcoholism. In the past the patient's behaviour was looked on as an expression of his moral turpitude. He might have been locked away in a Home for Inebriates for a year or more. Nowadays however emphasis is laid on the fact that from birth he has had a nervous system which is predisposed to addiction, if he indulges even in moderate amounts of alcohol. When the patient is well enough, he is encouraged to read a simple book which explains the new attitude to alcoholism (Williams, 1960).

(3) that at this stage it is a mistake to emphasise to the patient that he can never drink again. In favourable cases this realisation is likely to come later. One must remember that the patient's physical health will continue to improve during the succeeding weeks and months and as this takes place, he will be the better able to come to a firm decision about his future.

Apomorphine and disulfiram

In our experience this treatment should not be given to patients with severe disease of the liver or kidneys. It should also be withheld from those who have recently been on treatment with disulfiram (antabuse). Under these circumstances especially in the last case, there is a danger of a sudden advent of surgical shock, with a profound fall of blood pressure. For this reason the treatment should not be given unless there are facilities for (a) raising the foot of the bed, (b) giving insufflation with oxygen, and (c) injecting a stimulant such as nikethamide.

Apomorphine is given i.m. in a dose of 1/40 to 1/10 grain (1.5 to 6 mg). It is better later on to give 6 mg (1/10 grain) as it is a nuisance if not enough is given. After a few minutes the patient is likely to cough and also feel nauseated.

The patient is then given successive glasses of slightly warmed water flavoured by his favourite drink and thereafter vomits until his stomach is empty. He may have two or three successive spasms of vomiting, and in between, he is encouraged and almost forced to swallow the alcoholic drink. This need not be strong. It is the flavour which is important.

Some patients find this an extremely humiliating experience and for this reason emphasis is laid on the fact that they are doing something active themselves to effect their recovery.

During the treatment the patient is very suggestible and he is told that this treatment marks a change-over from being unable to control his drinking to actively disliking all alcoholic beverages.

The treatment has the following beneficial effects.

(1) The coughing and vomiting rids the patient of masses of mucus in the bronchi and stomach, so that he feels much better. (2) Whereas he has been physically tense before the treatment, the act of vomiting now relaxes him. (3) The drug is a sedative and the patient usually has a long sleep after the treatment. (4) Instead of thinking that his condition is hopeless, he feels that he has done something to help himself and he begins to have a picture in his mind of himself being restored to health. (5) This treatment can be repeated on six or seven occasions on alternate days, or if the patient is well enough on successive days. In either case he should have an addition of salt to his diet because of the amount lost in his vomitus. (6) The conditioning is often striking in its effects. We have

known a patient become severely nauseated when offered a drink, but such effects of course are merely temporary and serve only to give the patient a good start.

This treatment generally produces a remarkable change for the better in the patient's appearance and in his mood and expression.

We used to give atropine to terminate the session but in fact it does not diminish nausea. The nausea disappears rapidly if the patient is left in darkness and in complete quiet. He is likely to go to sleep for some hours. Contrariwise, if he is left in a bright and noisy ward his nausea will last for a considerable time. The best antidote is phenergan (25 mg i.m.).

This treatment can be supported by hypnosis as an adjunct to psychotherapy. The patient is given suggestions that he will recover under the new regime. At this stage the patient is subjected to group psychotherapy or he is visited by a member of Alcoholics Anonymous.

This organisation is particularly useful for patients who travel a great deal. They are given the addresses of secretaries of local branches throughout the world, so that they will not be without friends, in whatever country they find themselves.

An important drug in the treatment of alcoholism is disulfiram (antabuse). This is sold in tablets of 0.5 g. The tablets are scored, so that they can be broken into 2 or 4.

The drug is also available as a liquid, as some patients hide the tablet in their mouth and later dispose of it.

Under some regimes the patient is given a session in which he takes antabuse and thereafter he is given alcohol to drink. This is to show him what will happen if he drinks when on the drug. In our experience however this is unnecessary. The chief value of the drug is that if it is taken every morning at a fixed hour (generally when shaving before breakfast), this constitutes a ritual which reminds the patient that he is now living under a new regime. Under these circumstances it is not necessary to give the patient a high dose of the drug. We recommend 0.25 g for a week and after that 0.125 daily. This obviates anaemia or muscular twitchings or depression, and it also avoids severe complications, if the patient should have a relapse and drink to excess. It is still too early to assess the value of citrated calcium carbamate (temposil) said to be less toxic than antabuse.

It is generally advisable that the patient return to a different milieu from the previous one where he became ill. It is often advisable that he reports on the first of each month subsequently on his progress up to one year. (Paterson, 1950; Thompson, 1956; Wallerstein, 1957).

The Treatment of Drug Addiction

Addiction to opiates and to their synthetic substitutes is not such a problem in Great Britain as in America. However there has been some indication that owing to the severe measures taken against addicts in Canada, some of them are moving to England in order to profit from the conditions under the National Health Service.

There are mainly three types of addict. (1) Iatrogenic, where the patient has been given opiates for chronic or recurrent pain. (2) Unstable and tense individuals who have access to opiates. Addiction is an occupational hazard for physicians, nurses, pharmacists and merchant seamen among others. (3) Those in the entertainment world, such as musicians or pleasure-seekers, who are likely to encounter traffickers.

N-allylnormorphine

This is a remarkable antidote to morphine and also to its synthetic substitutes (Unna, 1943). It appears to act on the same sites as morphine, but displaces it. Its chief uses are (1) to help in rapidly diagnosing the degree of addiction. When an addict is injected with it, the degree of severity of the symptoms of withdrawal from morphine indicates the degree of dependence, a fact which otherwise might take a long time to discover. (2) Old patients who are given an injection of morphine may show an idiosyncrasy to the drug, and respiration may be depressed to a dangerous degree. This antidote will bring about immediate relief. (3) In obstetrics if the mother is injected with morphia, the foetal respiration may be dangerously depressed and an injection of the antidote may save its life. (4) In some parts of the world it is estimated that as many as 50 per cent of addicts attempt suicide by an overdose, in a final orgy. In such instances the drug may be life-saving. It is not, however, used for the treatment of the ordinary addict.

Institutional care

Unless the utmost precautions are taken, the chances of abstinence lasting for 5 years may be as low as 2 per cent (Wolff, 1945). Those who are treated by compulsion for 9 months show better results than voluntary patients. Factors in good prognosis are the comparatively short duration of addiction; cases where the original administration was for the relief of pain; good personality and high intelligence; interesting work; addiction to only one drug and that not heroin; a cycloid rather than an epileptoid temperament; rapid withdrawal (in one week); and where the drug has not been taken by injection.

Even where these conditions are favourable, however, the prognosis is still extremely grave and the patient should be sent whenever possible to an institution where the physician specialises in such cases.

The rate at which the drug should be withdrawn depends on the physical state of the patient and on the severity of the disorder.

If the addiction has been to heroin or if the daily dose of morphine has been high, it may be necessary to give methadone as a substitute, because it can be withdrawn more slowly. In this way the stress undergone by the patient is greatly reduced. One mg of methadone is said by Fraser and Grider (1953) to be equivalent to 4 mg of morphine, 2 mg of heroin, or 25 mg of pethidine or of codeine. The dose of the drug is then diminished by 50 per cent after 2 days and at 2 day intervals it is reduced to 30, 10 and 5 per cent of the amount which just prevents the appearance of symptoms of withdrawal. The moment which the patient dreads most is the first occasion on which no drug at all is given.

It is advisable that the same physician should treat the patient throughout.

No visitors are allowed, as they might bring drugs in, and care is taken by such devices as changing the patient's room while he is in a bath to make sure that he has no access to drugs which are hidden away.

We have mitigated the pain of withdrawal successfully by daily administration of ECT. Others use intramuscular paraldehyde or sodium amylobarbitone given by mouth. Nowadays librium or chlorpromazine are often employed.

We have been surprised how effective hypnosis can be for the treatment not only of addiction to barbiturates and alcohol, but even for a

References p. 221

combination of morphine and cocaine. Patients have reported that the symptoms of withdrawal become tolerable for some hours or days after induction of the hypnotic state.

In cases of marihuana or amphetamine, chlorpromazine is the most useful sedative during the period of diminishing the dose. With these drugs the symptoms of withdrawal are not so serious.

Psychotherapy and also the attainment of good physical health improve the prognosis. A change to an environment where the drug is not easily available is obviously desirable and contact with the treating physician should not be severed completely for a number of years.

The prognosis is by no means hopeless if every care is taken to give the patient the best available treatment, which practically always entails entering an institution for a time. For further reading, see Wolff (1945) and Paterson (1954).

The fact that drug addiction is low in the United Kingdom may be attributed to the attitude of the authorities to the problem. Addiction to a drug is considered more an illnes than a crime. In some parts of the world the attitude of the authorities to a drug addict is very severe. The view is taken that a great deal of crime is caused by drug addicts and they are treated as criminals of the worst sort. In England there are a number of addicts who go to their medical adviser, generally a psychiatrist, and obtain drugs by prescription. The addict nearly always cooperates in this treatment and the amount taken can often be cut down to a minimum. Theoretically one should aim at the ideal goal of getting the patient off the drug altogether. However, as Voltaire said, "the best can be the enemy of the good." The effects of opium and its derivatives in small doses are not incompatible with good health and there are a number of patients who are carrying on excellent work on small doses of the drug. Many of these people who are elderly are unable to face the mental stress of complete withdrawal. Even when this is attempted the results are not always satisfactory. In one case we attempted to take a medical mann off morphia. We were successful but the effect was that he had a very severe attack of gout following the withdrawal and after that he went into a state of hypomania which lasted some 18 months, after which he succumbed to a coronary thrombosis.

We always aim at persuading the patient to have a radical treatment for the addiction, but under certain circumstances we are content to cooperate with the patient, especially those in later life who have become accustomed to small doses of the drug. More recently, however, it has usually been possible to change the patient over to a drug less potent than morphia, and then wean him from that.

There is certainly a great gain from the point of view of the community in treating the addict as a patient rather than a criminal.

Conclusion

There is general agreement that the advent of psychotropic drugs has been of immense benefit in treating mental disorders. The phenothiazines in particular have calmed the excited and deluded patient and made him accessible to psychotherapy and rehabilitation. The anti-depressive drugs such as imipramine, amitriptyline and the MAOI's have acted not merely temporarily on symptoms, as the amphetamines do, but in a more radical and lasting manner on the behaviour pattern. The main drawback however of this class is their toxicity, especially the MAOI's, and their slowness to take effect. Again, the minor tranquillisers, especially librium, have proved a useful addition to our pharmacopoeia. Their forerunners, the barbiturates, though of immense value, tend to cause drowsiness, when used as sedatives, and when used as soporifics they can cause addiction, with the all-too-common periodic overdose. It is well to be acquainted with possible alternatives both for sedation and for the production of sleep.

Another development has been the use of psychotogenic drugs like lysergic acid diethyl-amide. Hitherto the psychiatrist has been able merely to describe the subjective sensations of mental patients. Now however it is possible to study symptoms such as hallucinations under experimental conditions. Under the conditions of the "model" or artificially produced "psychosis", the subjective symptoms can be correlated with alterations in the EEG, as studied by the newer methods. The same drugs, however, when considered as psycholytic or abreactive agents, should be employed only by experts. Although the probing of early memories is a dramatic procedure, it is doubtful if the danger involved justifies the risk. Many believe that equally satisfactory results can be obtained by simpler procedures such as giving a combination of sodium amylobarbitone and methedrine. This is a safer method when abreactive therapy is indicated.

There still remains some uneasiness on the part of psychiatrists regarding the misuse of psychotropic drugs. There is a feeling that psychotherapy and occupational therapy are "natural" procedures but that electrical and drug treatments are "unnatural". However the psychiatrist is apt to resort to these measures only in those cases where other methods fail, just as one resorts to surgery when the patient is beyond medical care. As in the case of the surgeon, the neuropsychiatrist must be experienced in his specialty. It is to be hoped that the information given in this book will help the reader further to give these specialised treatments to the right patients and in the correct manner.

The advent of psychopharmacology has indeed made a considerable impact on the attitude of the average psychiatrist towards mental illness. Wikler (1957), Garattini and Ghetti (1957), Lewis (1959), Uhr and Miller (1960), Delay and Deniker (1960), Kalinowsky and Hoch (1961) and Rothlin (1961) have shown that the administration of drugs can cause marked changes in feeling and behaviour which are of a more differentiated and refined character than have hitherto been possible. Pharmacology has drawn attention away from the purely subjective approach to the patient and directed it to the study of brain function. This approach is al so being made in oher forms of treatment besides the administration of drugs. These consist chiefly of stress treatments, including ECT, conditioning methods, abreactive treatment, hypnosis and autogenic training or (for the more intractable conditions) brain surgery.

The study of the physiology of the brain and nervous system has been greatly facilitated by new techniques in electroencephalography. Progress is being made in the study of the emotional and behavioural reactions of normal and abnormal individuals to certain pre-arranged situations including conditioning. One can study such functions as the heart-beat, the electrical skin reaction (psychogalvanic reflex) and respiration. Again, the way in which the brain responds to conditioned and unconditioned stimuli has now been demonstrated much more clearly since the introduction of the method of averaging many responses to a stimulus by means of an electronic computer (Brazier, 1962) or by the use of a simpler and less expensive device (Spinelli and Paterson, 1962).

By such methods the psychiatrist is likely to move onwards from the present era of empiricism to one in which cerebral mechanisms are better understood.

References p. 221

References to Part II

ABRAMSON, H. A. (1957), Verbatim recording and transference studies with lysergic acid diethylamide (L.S.D.-25), *J. nerv. ment. Dis.*, 125, 444.

ALEXANDER, L. (1961 a), Effects of psychotropic drugs on conditional responses in man, in: *Neuropsychopharmacology*, E. ROTHLIN (Ed.), Elsevier, Amsterdam.

ALEXANDER, L. (1961 b), Objective evaluation of antidepressant therapy by conditional reflex technique, *Dis. nerv. Syst.*, 22 (5) (Sect. 2, Suppl.), p. 14.

AMBROSIO, A. (1957), Risultati dello studio oftalmoscopico di un gruppo di soggetti sottoposti a trattamento clorpromazinico, *Ann. Ophthalm.*, 83, 588.

AMERICAN MEDICAL ASSOCIATION, COUNCIL ON DRUGS (1959), *New and nonofficial drugs*, J. B. Lippincott, Philadelphia.

ANNESLEY, P. T. AND MANT, A. K. (1962), A fatal reaction to thioproperazine, *Brit. med. J.*, 1, 233.

ANSTREICHER, K. (1960), Fatalities during or following fluphenazine therapy, *Delaware med. J.*, 32, 430.

ARMITAGE, P. (1950), Sequential analysis with more than two alternative hypotheses, and its relation to discriminant function analysis, *J. R. statist. Soc.*, 12, 137.

ARNOLD, O. H., HIFT. S. AND HOFF, H. (1960), Die Stellung der psychotropen Drogen im Gesamtbehandlungsplan der Psychiatrie, *Wien. med. Wschr.*, 110, 238.

AYD, F. J., JR. (1957), Treatment of ambulatory and hospitalized psychiatric patients with trilafon, *Dis. nerv. Syst.*, 18, 394.

AYD, F. J., JR. (1960 a), *Neuroleptics and extrapyramidal reactions*, in: *Extrapyramidal system and neuroleptics*, J. M. BORDELEAU (Ed.), Editions Psychiatriques, Montreal, p. 355.

AYD, F. J., JR. (1960 b), The current status of major anti-depressants, *American Psychiatric Association, District Branch*, Publication No. 1, Feb., Washington, D.C., pp. 213-222.

AYD, F. J., JR. (1961 a), A critique of antidepressants, *Dis. nerv. Syst.*, 22, No. 5, Sect. 2, Suppl. p. 32.

AYD, F. J., JR. (1961 b), Toxic somatic and psychopathologic reactions to antidepressant drugs, *J. Neuropsychiat.*, 2, Suppl. 1, p. 119.

AZIMA, H., DUROST, H. AND ARTHURS, D. (1960), The effect of R-1625 (Haloperidol) in mental syndromes: a multiblind study, *Amer. J. Psychiat.*, 117, 546.

BAIRD, I. M. AND BUCKLER, J. W. (1962), Clinical trial of methaqualone as a hypnotic, *Practitioner*, 188, 361.

BALL, J. R. B. AND KILOH, L. G. (1959), A controlled trial of imipramine in treatment of depressive states, *Brit. med. J.*, 2, 1052.

BAMBACE, F. (1961), Effects of chlordiazepoxide in severely disturbed outpatients, *Amer. J. Psychiat.*, 118, 69.

BARDONI, F. (1960), Sul trattamento di ammalati mentali con il 2-cloro-9 – (3′ dimetil-amino-propilidene) – tioxantine. Nota clinica, *Rass. Studi psichiat.*, 49, 608.

BARRON, A., BECKENNG, B., RUDY, L. H. AND SMITH, J. A. (1961), A double blind study comparing R04-0403, trifluoperazine and a placebo in chronically ill mental patients, *Amer. J. Psychiat.*, 118, 347.

BARSA, J. A. AND KLINE, N. S. (1955), Combined reserpine-chlorpromazine therapy in disturbed psychotics, *Amer. J. Psychiat.*, 111, 780.

BARSA, J. A. AND SAUNDERS, J. C. (1961), Fluphenazine: use with chronic psychotic patients, *Dis. nerv. Syst.*, 22, 211.

BARUK, H. AND LAUNAY, J. (1961), La loi des stades et la pharmacologie expérimen-tale chez le singe, in: E. ROTHLIN (Ed.), *Neuropsychopharmacology*, Vol. 2, Else-vier, Amsterdam.

BATES, T. J. N. AND DOUGLAS, A. D. M. (1961), A comparative trial of four monoamine oxidase inhibitors on chronic depressives, *J. ment. Sci.*, 107, 538.

BATTERMAN, R. C., GROSSMAN, A. J., LEIFER, P. AND MOURATOFF, G. J. (1959), Clinical re-evaluation of daytime sedatives, *Postgrad. Med.*, 26, 502.

BECKER, A. M. (1949), Zur Psychopathologie der Lysergsäurediäthylamidwirkung, *Wien. Z. Nervenheilk.*, 2, 402.

BECKMAN, H. (1961), *Pharmacology: the nature, action and use of drugs*, 2nd Edition, W. B. Saunders, Philadelphia.

BEECH, H. R., DAVIES, B. M. AND MORGENSTERN, F. S. (1961), Preliminary investigations of the effects of sernyl upon cognitive and sensory processes, *J. ment. Sci.*, 107, 509.

BEECHER, H. K. (1955), The powerful placebo, *J. Amer. med. Ass.*, 159, 1602.

BENNETT, I. F. (1959), Clinical studies with phenothiazine derivatives in psychiatry, *Res. Publ. Ass. nerv. ment. Dis.*, 37, 266.

BERGER, F. M. (1960), *Classification of psychoactive drugs according to their chemical structures and sites of action*, in: *Drugs and Behavior*, L. UHR and J. G. MILLER (Eds.), John Wiley & Sons, New York, p. 86.

BERGER, F. M. AND BRADLEY, W. (1946), The pharmacological properties of $\alpha : \beta$ dihydroxy-γ – (2-methylphenoxy) – propane (myanesin), *Brit. J. Pharmacol.*, 1, 265.

BIRD, C. E. (1960), Agranulocytosis due to imipramine (tofranil), *Canad. med. Ass. J.*, 82, 1021.

BLAIR, D. (1960), Treatment of severe depression by imipramine (tofranil) an investi-gation of 100 cases, *J. ment. Sci.*, 106, 905.

BOBON, J. AND COLLARD, J. (1962), Un neuroleptique original à effet hypnogène différé: le R 3345 ou dipiperon, *Compt. rend. congr. psychiat. neurol. Lang. franç.*, Mont-pellier, 59, 538.

BOITTELLE, G. AND BOITTELLE-LENTULO, C. (1959), A propos d'un nouveau neuroplégi-que, le Ro. 04.403, *Ann. méd.-psychol.*, 117 (ii), 515.

BRODIE, B. B., SULSER, S. AND COSTA, E. (1960), *Theories on mechanism of action of psychotropic drugs*, in: *Extrapyramidal system and neuroleptics*, J. M. BORDELEAU (Ed.), Editions Psychiatriques, Montreal, p. 183.

BRADLEY, P. B., DENIKER, P. AND RADOUCO-THOMAS, C. (Eds.), (1959), *Neuropsycho-pharmacology*, Vol. 1, Elsevier, Amsterdam.

BRANDRUP, E. AND KRISTJANSEN, P. (1961), A controlled clinical test of a new psycho-leptic drug (Haloperidol), *J. ment. Sci.*, 107, 778.

BRAZIER, M. A. B. (1962), The analysis of brain waves, *Sci. American*, 206, 142.

BRITISH MEDICAL JOURNAL (1960), To-day's drugs: methaminodiazepoxide, 2, 797.

BROUSSOLLE, P., PERRIN, J., MAUREL, P., LAMBERT, P. A., ACHAINTRE, A., BALVET, P.,

BEAUJARD, M., REVOL, L., REQUET, A. AND BERTHIER, C., (1957), La prochloperazine en psychiatrie; expérience tirée de 240 cures, *Presse méd.*, 65, 1628.

BRUCE, E. M., *et al.* (1960), A comparative trial of E.C.T. and tofranil, *Amer. J. Psychiat.*, 117, 76.

BUSCH, A. K. AND JOHNSON, W. C. (1950), L.S.D. 25 as an aid in psychotherapy (preliminary report of a new drug), *Dis. nerv. Syst.*, 11, 241.

CAHN, C. H. AND LEHMANN, H. E. (1957), Perphenazine; observations on the clinical effects of a new tranquillizing agent in psychotic conditions, *Canad. psychiat. Ass. J.*, 2, 104.

CAHN, M. M. AND LEVY, E. J. (1957), Ultraviolet light factor in chlorpromazine dermatitis, *A. M. A. Arch. Derm.*, 75, 38.

CALDWELL, A. E. (1958), *Psychopharmaca: a bibliography of psychopharmacology (1952-57)*, U.S. Department of Health, Education and Welfare, Washington, D.C., p. 33.

CARSTAIRS, G. M. (1961), Advances in psychological medicine, *Practitioner*, 187, 495.

CASEY, J. F., LASKY, J. J., KLETT, C. J. AND HOLLISTER, L.-E. (1960 a), Treatment of schizophrenic reactions with phenothiazine derivatives. A comparative study of chlorpromazine, triflupromazine, mepazine, prochlorperazine, perphenazine and phenobarbital, *Amer. J. Psychiat.*, 117, 97.

CASEY, J. F., *et al.* (1960 b), Drug therapy in schizophrenia: a controlled study of the relative effectiveness of chlorpromazine, promazine, phenobarbital, and placebo, *A. M. A. Arch. gen. Psychiat.*, 2, 210.

CASEY, J. F., HOLLISTER, L. E., KLETT, C. J., LASKEY, J. J. AND CAFFEY, E. M., JR. (1961), Combined drug therapy of chronic schizophrenics. Controlled evaluation of placebo, dextro-amphetamine, imipramine, isocarboxazid an trifluoperazine added to maintenance doses of chlorpromazine, *Amer. J. Psychiat.*, 117, 997.

CHILDERS, R. T., JR. (1961), Controlling the chronically disturbed patient with massive phenothiazine therapy, *Amer. J. Psychiat.*, 118, 246.

COHEN, S. (1960), Lysergic acid diethylamide: side effects and complications, *J. nerv. ment. Dis.*, 130, 30.

COHEN, S., FISCHMAN, L. AND EISHER, B. G. (1958), Subjective reports of lysergic acid experiences in a context of psychological test performance, *Amer. J. Psychiat.*, 115, 30.

COLE, J. O., GONEZ, R. T. AND KLERMAN, G. L. (1961), Drug therapy, *Progr. Neurol. Psychiat.*, 16, 539.

COLLARD, J. (1960), *Psychopharmacologie comparée du haloperidol et de ses dérivés (tripéridol, methylpéridide, "R-1647")*, in: J. M. BORDELEAU (Ed.), *Extrapyramidal system and neuroleptics*, Editions Psychiatriques, Montreal, p. 369.

CONDRAU, G. (1949), Klinische Erfahrungen an Geisteskranken mit Lysergsäurediäthyl- amid, *Acta psychiat. (Kbh.)*, 24, 9.

CONN, H. (1961), *Current therapy*, W. B. Saunders, Philadelphia.

CONNELL, P. H. (1958), *Amphetamine psychosis*, Chapman and Hall, London.

CRAMOND, W. A. (1962), Thioproperazine, *Lancet*, 1, 592.

CUTNER, M. (1959), Analytic work with L.S.D. 25, *Psychiat. Quart.*, 33, 715.

DARLING, H. F. (1961), Chlorprothixene (taractan) and isocarboxazid (marplan) in psychotic depressions, *Amer. J. Psychiat.*, 117, 31.

DAVIES, B. M. (1960), A preliminary report on the use of sernyl in psychiatric illness, *J. ment. Sci.*, 106, 1073.

DAVIES, B. M. AND BEECH, H. R. (1960), The effect of sernyl on twelve normal volunteers, *J. ment. Sci.*, 106, 912.

De Giacomo, U. (1951), Les catatonies toxiques experimentales, *Acta neurol. (Napoli)*, 6, 5.

De Jong, H. (1945), *Experimental catatonia*, Williams & Wilkins, Baltimore.

Delay, J. and Deniker, P. (1960), *Apport de la clinique à la connaissance de l'action des neuroleptiques*, in: *Extrapyramidal system and neuroleptics*, J. M. Bordeleau (Ed.), Editions Psychiatriques, Montreal, p. 301.

Delay, J. and Deniker, P. (1961), *Méthodes chimiothérapiques en psychiatrie: les nouveaux médicaments psychotropes*, Masson et Cie, Paris.

Delay, J., Deniker, P. and Hart, J. M. (1952), Utilisation en thérapeutique psychiatrique d'une phenothiazine d'action centrale élective, *Ann. méd.-psychol.*, Par., 110 (2) 112.

Delay, J., Pichot, P., Lempérière, T. and Elissalde, B. (1960), Halopéridol et chimiothérapie des psychoses, *Presse méd.*, 68, 1353.

Denber, H. C. B., Rajotte, P. and Ross, E. (1960), Some observations on the chemotherapy of depression: results with "taractan", *Comprehens. Psychiat.*, 1, 308.

Denham, J. and Carrick, D. J. E. L. (1961), Therapeutic value of thioproperazine and the importance of the associated neurological disturbances, *J. ment. Sci.*, 107, 326.

Dorfman, W. (1961), Masked depression, *Dis. nerv. Syst.*, 22 (5), Pt. 2, 41.

Ellsworth, R. B. and Clayton, W. H. (1959), Measurement of improvement in "mental illness", *J. cons. Psychol.*, 23, 15.

English, D. C. (1961), A comparative study of antidepressants in balanced therapy, *Amer. J. Psychiat.*, 117, 865.

English, H. L. (1959), An alarming side-effect of tofranil, *Lancet*, 1, 1231.

Essig, C. F. and Ainslie, J. D. (1957), Addiction to meprobamate, *J. Amer. med. Ass.*, 164, 1382.

Extra Pharmacopoeia (1958), 24th Edition, The Pharmaceutical Press, London. Also *Supplement* (1961).

Fabing, H. O. and Hawkins, J. R. (1956), A year's experience with frenquel in clinical and experimental schizophrenic psychoses, *Dis. nerv. Syst.*, 16, 329.

Feer, H., Fuchs, M. and Strässle, M. (1960), Klinische Untersuchungen mit Chlorprothixen (Taractan), *Schweiz. med. Wschr.*, 90, 600.

Feldman, P. E. (1961), Psychotherapy and chemotherapy (amitriptyline) of anergic states, *Dis. nerv. Syst.*, 22, No. 5, Sect. 2 – Suppl. p. 27.

Fischer, R., Georgi, F. and Weber, R. (1951), Psychophysische Korrelationen: Modellversuche zum Schizophrenieproblem Lysergsäurediäthylamid und Mescalin, *Schweiz. med. Wschr.*, 81, 817 and 837.

Fisher, R. A. (1950), *Statistical methods for research workers*, 11th ed. Oliver & Boyd, Edinburgh and London, p. 211.

Fleminger, J. J. and Groden, B. M. (1962), Clinical features of depression and response to imipramine (Tofranil), *J. ment. Sci.*, 108, 101.

Folkard, M. S. (1957), *A sociological contribution to the understanding of aggression and its treatment in a mental hospital*, Ph. D. Thesis, Univ. London.

Fraser, H. F. and Grider, J. A., Jr. (1953), Treatment of drug addiction, *Amer. J. Med.*, 14, 571.

Freeman, H., Kenefick, D. P. and Rivera, M. R. (1960), A clinical evaluation of marplan in depressed patients, *Dis. nerv. Syst.*, 21, No. 3, Sect. 2 – Suppl. p. 104.

Freud, S. (1933), *New introductory lectures on psycho-analysis*, W. W. Norton & Co., New York, p. 211.

FREYHAN, F. A. (1961 a), *The influence of specific and non-specific factors on the clinical effects of psychotropic drugs*, in: *Neuropsychopharmacology*, E. ROTHLIN (Ed.), Elsevier, Amsterdam, p. 189.

FREYHAN, F. A. (1961 b), Loss of ejaculation during mellaril treatment, *Amer. J. Psychiat.*, 118, 171.

GARATTINI, S. AND GHETTI, V. (1957), *Psychotropic drugs*, Elsevier, Amsterdam.

GARRY, J. W. AND LEONARD, T. J. (1962), Haloperidol: a controlled trial in chronic schizophrenia, *J. ment. Sci.*, 108, 105.

GELLER, W. (1960), Therapeutische Ergebnisse mit dem Neurolepticum Truxal, *Med. Klin.*, 55, 554.

GOLDMAN, D. (1959), Clinical experience with newer antidepressant drugs and some related electroencephalographic observations, *Ann. N.Y. Acad. Sci.*, 80, 687.

GOLDMAN, D. (1960), *Parkinsonism and related phenomena from administration of drugs: their production and control under clinical conditions and possible relation to therapeutic effect*, in: *Extrapyramidal system and neuroleptics*, J. M. BORDELEAU (Ed.), Editions Psychiatriques, Montreal.

GOOSZEN, J. A. H. (1961), Psychopharmacologic agents: pathophysiological considerations, *Psychiat. Neurol. Neurochir. (Amst.)*, 64, 257.

GREEN, F. H. K. (1954), The clinical evaluation of remedies, *Lancet*, 2, 1085.

GROSS, M., HITCHMAN, I. C., REEVES, W. P., LAWRENCE, J. AND NEWELL, P. C. (1961), *Discontinuation of treatment with ataractic drugs*, in: *Recent Advances in Biological Psychiatry*, J. WORTIS (Ed.), Vol. 3, Grune and Stratton, New York, p. 44.

HARAN, T. (1960), Perphenazine (fentazin) in the management of chronic schizophrenia, *J. Irish med. Ass.*, 46, 135.

HARE, E. H., DOMINIAN, J. AND SHARPE, L. (1962), Phenelzine and dexamphetamine in depressive illness: a comparative trial, *Brit. med. J.*, 1, 9.

HARGREAVES, M. A. (1959), An investigation into the effects of azacyclonal on the hallucinations of chronic schizophrenic patients, *J. ment. Sci.*, 105, 210.

HARRIS, J. A. AND ROBIN, A. A. (1960), A controlled study of phenelzine in depressive reactions, *J. ment. Sci.*, 106, 1432.

HAYDU, G. G., BRINITZER, W., GIBBON, J. AND GOLDSCHMIDT, L. (1961), A clinical trial with chlorprothixene (taractan), *Amer. J. Psychiat.*, 118, 460.

HIMWICH, H. E. (1960), *Biochemical and neurophysiological action of psychoactive drugs*, in: *Drugs and Behavior*, L. UHR and J. G. MILLER (Eds.), John Wiley & Sons, New York, p. 41.

HINES, L. R. (1960), Methaminodiazepoxide (librium): A psychotherapeutic drug, *Curr. ther. Res.*, 2, 227.

HOCH, P. H. (1959), *Pharmacologically induced psychoses*, in: *American Handbook of Psychiatry*, S. ARIETI (Ed.), Basic Books, New York, p. 1703.

HOFMANN, A., FREY, A., OTT, H., PETRZILKA, T. AND TROXLER, F. (1958), Konstitutionsaufklärung und Synthese von Psilocybin, *Experientia (Basel)*, 14, 397.

HOLLIDAY, A. R., DUFFY, M. C. AND DILLE, J. M. (1958), The effects of certain tranquillizers on a stress producing behavioral task, *J. Pharmacol. exp. Ther.*, 122, 32 A.

HOLLISTER, L. E., MOTZENBECKER, F. P. AND DEGAN, R. O. (1961), Withdrawal reactions from chlordiazepoxide ("librium"), *Psychopharmacologia (Berl.)*, 2, 63.

HOLT, J. P. AND WRIGHT, E. R. (1960), Preliminary results with fluphenazine (prolixin) in chronic psychotic patients, *Amer. J. Psychiat.*, 117, 157.

HOLT, J. P., WRIGHT, E. R. AND HECKER, A. O. (1960), Comparative clinical experience with five antidepressants, *Amer. J. Psychiat.*, 117, 533.

HORSLEY, J. S. (1936), Narcoanalysis, *J. ment. Sci.*, 82, 416.

HUTCHINSON, J. T. AND SMEDBERG, D. (1960), Phenelzine ("nardil") in the treatment of endogenous depression, *J. ment. Sci.*, 106, 704.

IMLAH, N. W. (1960), Overshooting action of phenelzine, *Lancet*, 1, 826.

ISBELL, H. (1959), Comparison of the reactions induced by psilocybin and lsd-25 in man, *Psychopharmacologia (Berl.)*, 1, 29.

JACKSON, E. B. (1961), Mellaril in the treatment of the geriatric patient, *Amer. J. Psychiat.*, 118, 543.

JENNER, F. A., KERRY, R. J. AND PARKIN, D. (1961), A controlled comparison of methaminodiazepoxide (chlordiazepoxide, "librium") and amylobarbitone in the treatment of anxiety in neurotic patients, *J. ment. Sci.*, 107, 583.

JOSHI, V. G. (1961), Controlled clinical trial of isocarboxazid ("marplan") in hospital psychiatry, *J. ment. Sci.*, 107, 567.

KALINOWSKY, L. B. AND HOCH, P. H. (1961), *Somatic treatments in psychiatry*, 3rd Edit., Grune and Stratton, New York.

KANJILAL, G. C. AND MATHESON, B. (1962), A trial tetrabenazine in disturbed mentally subnormal patients, *J. ment. Sci.*, 108, 225.

KEMP, W., APOLITO, A., OLINGEN, L., SCHWARTZ, M. AND YACHNES, E. (1960), Tofranil (imipramine) in the treatment of depressive states, *J. nerv. ment. Dis.*, 130, 146.

KENNEDY, A. (1961), The use of anti-depressant drugs, *J. ment. Sci.*, 107, 989.

KILLAM, E. K. AND KILLAM, K. F. (1957), *The influence of drugs on central afferent pathways*, in: *Brain Mechanisms and Drug Action*, W. S. FIELDS (Ed.), C. C. Thomas, Springfield, Ill., p. 71.

KILOH, L. G. AND BALL, J. R. B. (1961), Depression treated with imipramine: a follow-up study, *Brit. med. J.*, 1, 168.

KING, P. D. (1959), Phenelzine and E.C.T. in the treatment of depressions, *Amer. J. Psychiat.*, 116, 64.

KINROSS-WRIGHT, J. V. (1955), *Discussion on medical and other measures to be taken to keep the discharged patient from returning to the institution*, in: *Chlorpromazine and Mental Health*, Proceedings of the symposium held under the auspices of Smith, Kline and French Laboratories. Lea & Febiger, Philadelphia, p. 154.

KINROSS-WRIGHT, J. V. (1959), Newer phenothiazine drugs in treatment of nervous disorders, *J. Amer. med. Ass.*, 170, 1283.

KINROSS-WRIGHT, J. V., COHEN, I. M. AND KNIGHT, J. A. (1960), The management of neurotic and psychotic states with Ro 5-0690 (librium), *Dis. nerv. Syst.*, 21, No. 3, Sect 2 – Suppl. p. 23.

KLINE, N. S. (1961), Comprehensive therapy of depression, *J. Neuropsychiat.*, 2, Suppl. 1, p. 15.

KNIGHT, J. A. (1961), Drug-induced hepatic injury: marplan hepatitis, *Amer. J. Psychiat.*, 118, 73.

KRIS, E. B. (1961), *Effects of pharmacotherapy on work and learning ability – a five year follow–up study*, J. WORTIS (Ed.), *Recent Advances in Biological Psychiatry*, Vol. 3, Grune and Stratton, New York, p. 30.

KRISTJANSEN, P., BORUP SVENDSEN, B. AND FAURBYE, A. (1962), Etude comparative contrôlée de l'effet de la thioridazine et de la chlorpromazine dans la schizophrénie chronique, *Compt. rend. congrès psychiat. neurol. Lang. franç.*, Montpellier, 59, 518.

KRUSE, W. (1960), Treatment of drug-induced extrapyramidal symptoms, *Dis. nerv. Syst.*, 21, 8.

KUHN, R. (1957), Über die Behandlung depressiver Zustande mit einem Iminodibenzylderivat (G 22355), *Schweiz. med. Wschr.*, 87, 1135.

KUHN, R. (1960), Probleme der praktischen Durchführung der Tofranil-Behandlung, *Wien. med. Wschr.*, 110, 245.

KURLAND, A. A. (1957), The drug placebo – its psychodynamic and conditional reflex action, *Behav. Sci.*, 2, 101.

LABORIT, H., HUGUENARD, P. AND ALLUAUME, R. (1952), Un nouveau stabilisateur végétatif: le 4560 rp, *Presse méd.*, 60, 20.

LA BROSSE, E. H., AXELROD, J. AND KETY, S. S. (1958), O-methylation, the principal route of metabolism of epinephrine in man, *Science*, 128, 593.

LANCASTER, N. P. AND FOSTER, A. R. (1959), Suicidal attempt by imipramine overdosage, *Brit. med. J.*, 2, 1458.

LANCET (1961), Annotation, "Thioproperazine", *Lancet*, 2, 698.

LANCET (1962), Leading Article, Thalidomide and congenital malformations, *Lancet*, I, 307.

LA VERNE, A. A. (1961a), Compendium of neuropsychopharmacology, *J. Neuropsychiat.*, 3, 127.

LA VERNE, A. A. (1961b), Compendium of neuropsychopharmacology, *J. Neuropsychiat.*, 3, 197.

LEHMANN, H. E., CAHN, C. H. AND DE VERTEUIL, R. L. (1958), The treatment of depressive conditions with imipramine (G 22355), *Canad. psychiat. Ass. J.*, 3, 155.

LEWIS, A. (1959), in: P. B. BRADLEY, P. DENIKER AND C. RADOUCO-THOMAS (Eds.), *Neuropsychopharmacology*, Vol. 1, Elsevier, Amsterdam, p. 207.

LOOMER, H. P., SAUNDERS, J. C. AND KLINE, N. S. (1957), A clinical and pharmacodynamic evaluation of iproniazid as a psychic energizer, *Psychiat. Res. Rep. Amer. Psychiat. Ass.*, No. 8, p. 129.

LORR, M. (1960), *Rating scales, behavior inventories, and drugs*, in: *Drugs and Behavior*, L. UHR and J. G. MILLER (Eds.), John Wiley & Sons, New York, p. 519.

LUBY, E. D., COHEN, B. D., ROSENBAUM, G., GOTTLIEB, J. S. AND KELLY, R. (1959), Study of a new schizophrenomimetic drug – sernyl, *A. M. A. Arch. Neurol. Psychiat.*, 81, 363.

LUKE, E. AND WYLLIE, J. H. (1961), Thioproperazine, *Lancet*, 2, 720.

LURIE, M. L. AND SALZER, H. M. (1961), Tranylcypromine (parnate) in the ambulatory treatment of depressed patients, *Amer. J. Psychiat.*, 118, 152.

MACDONALD, R. AND WATTS, T. P. SHIELDS (1959), Trifluoperazine dihydrochloride ("stelazine") in paranoid schizophrenia, *Brit. med. J.*, 1, 549.

MCILWAIN, H. (1959), *Biochemistry and the central nervous system*, 2nd Edit., Churchill, London.

MCNEILL, D. L. M. AND MADGWICK, J. R. A. (1961), A comparison of results in schizophrenics treated with (1) insulin, (2) trifluoperazine ("stelazine"), *J. ment. Sci.*, 107, 297.

MALAMUD, W., BARTON, W. E., FLEMING, A. M., MIDDLETON, P. McK., FRIEDMAN, T. T. AND SCHLEIFER, M. J. (1957), The evaluation of the effects of derivatives of rauwolfia in the treatment of schizophrenia, *Amer. J. Psychiat.*, 114, 193.

MALITZ, S. AND HOCH, P. H. (1956), Preliminary evaluation of new phenothiazine derivative, N.P. 207, *Psychiat. Quart.*, 30, 633.

MARLEY, E. (1959), Response to drugs in psychiatry, *J. ment. Sci.*, 105, 19.

MARQUIS, D. G., KELLY, E. L., MILLER, J. G., GERARD, R. W. AND RAPOPORT, A. (1957), Experimental studies of behavioral effects of meprobamate on normal subjects, *Ann. N. Y. Acad. Sci.*, 67, 701.

MARTIN, A. J. (1957), L.S.D. (lysergic acid diethylamide) treatment of chronic psycho-neurotic patients under day-hospital conditions, *Int. J. Soc. Psychiat.*, 3, 188.

MATÉFI, L. (1952), Mescalin- und Lysergsäurediäthylamid-Rausch, *Confin. neurol. (Basel)*, 12, 146.

MAY, R. H., SELEYNES, E., WEEKLEY, R. D. AND COX, A. M. (1960), Thioridazine therapy: results and complications, *J. nerv. ment. Dis.*, 130, 230.

MEDUNA, L. J. (1950), *Carbon dioxide therapy*, C. C. Thomas, Springfield, Ill.

MEYLER, L. (1960), *Side effects of drugs*, Excerpta Medica Foundation, Amsterdam, p. 13.

MIDDLEFELL, R., FROST, I., EGAN, G. P. AND EATON, H. (1960), A report on the effects of phenelzine (nardil) a monoamine oxidase inhibitor, in depressed patients, *J. ment. Sci.*, 106, 1533.

MILLER, A., BAKER, E. F. W., LEWIS, D. AND JONES, A. (1960), Imipramine, a clinical evaluation in a variety of settings, *Canad. psychiat. Ass. J.*, 5, 150.

MILNE, H. B. AND FOWLER, D. B. (1960), A clinical trial of largactil stemetil and veractil (nozinan), *J. ment. Sci.*, 106, 1105.

MORIARTY, J. D. (1959), Broad spectrum treatment of the neurotic and the borderline psychotic patient in office practice, *J. Neuropsychiat.*, 1, 112.

MORROW, L. E. (1961), Fluphenazine in private psychiatric practice, *Amer. J. Psychiat.*, 117, 1031.

MÜLLER, J. M., SCHITTLER, E. AND BEIN, H. J. (1952), Reserpin, der sedative Wirk-stoff aus Rauwolfia Serpentina Benth, *Experientia*, 8, 338.

MUNSTER, A. J., STANLEY, A. M. AND SAUNDERS, J. C. (1961), Imipramine (tofranil) in the treatment of enuresis, *Amer. J. Psychiat.*, 118, 76.

NIELSEN, I. M. AND NEUHOLD, K. (1959), The comparative pharmacology and toxicology of the transisomer of 2-chloro-9-(3'-dimethylaminopropylidene)-thiaxanthene, HCl (chlorprothixene) = n 714 trans and chlorpromazine, *Acta pharmacol. (Kbh.)*, 15, 335.

OLTMAN, J. E. AND FRIEDMAN, S. (1961 a), Preliminary report on taractan, *Amer. J. Psychiat.*, 117, 1120.

OLTMAN, J. E. AND FRIEDMAN, S. (1961 b), Elavil in the treatment of affective dis-orders (and comparison with tofranil), *Amer. J. Psychiat.*, 118, 546.

PAREDES, A., GOGERTY, J. H. AND WEST, L. J. (1961), Psychopharmacology, *Curr. psychiat. Ther.*, 1, 54.

PATERSON, A. S. (1950), Modern techniques for the treatment of acute and prolonged alcoholism, *Brit. J. Addict.*, 47, No. 2, p. 3.

PATERSON, A. S. (1954), Addiction to morphia and allied drugs: some recent develop-ments, *Postgrad. med. J.*, 30, 622.

PATERSON, A. S., PASSERINI, D., BRACCHI, F. AND BLACK, S. (1962), L'hypnose et l'action de drogues ataractiques étudiée par la méthode du reflexe conditionné chez l'homme, *Compt. rend. congrès psychiat. neurol. Lang. franç.*, Montpellier, 1961, p. 336.

PAULSON, G. (1960), Procyclidine for dystonia caused by phenothiazine derivatives, *Dis. nerv. Syst.*, 21, 447.

POELDINGER, W. (1960), Ein Neurolepticum mit antidepressiver Wirkung, Taractan (Ro 4-0403), *Praxis*, 49, 468.

PRESSMAN, M. D. AND WEISS, L. B. (1961), Experiences with elavil: treatment of fifty-one cases of depression, *Amer. J. Psychiat.*, 118, 74.

PRESTON, J. B. (1956), Effects of chlorpromazine on the central nervous system of the cat: a possible neural basis for action, *J. Pharmacol. exp. Ther.*, 118, 100.

RATHOD, N. H. (1958), Tranquillisers and patient's environment, *Lancet*, 1, 611.

RATHOD, N. H. (1961), Experience with promazine, *Amer. J. Psychiat.*, 118, 504.

RAVN, J. (1961), Chlorprothixene: a new psychotropic entity, *Amer. J. Psychiat.*, 118, 227.

REES, L. AND DAVIES, B. (1961), A controlled trial of phenelzine ("nardil") in the treatment of severe depressive illness, *J. ment. Sci.*, 107, 560.

REES, W. L. AND LAMBERT, C. (1955), The value and limitations of chlorpromazine in the treatment of anxiety states, *J. ment. Sci.*, 101, 834.

REMY, M. (1958), Essai d'un nouveau dérivé de la phénothiazine, le melléril, en clinique psychiatrique, *Schweiz. med. Wschr.*, 88, 1221.

REZNIKOFF, L. (1961), The use of fluphenazine (prolixen) in rehabilitation of chronic schizophrenic patients, *Amer. J. Psychiat.*, 117, 457.

RICHTER, C. P. AND PATERSON, A. S. (1932), Pharmacology of the grasp reflex, *Brain*, 55, 391.

RICKELS, K., CLARK, T. W., EWING, J. H., KLINGENSMITH, W. C., MORRIS, H. M. AND SMOCK, C. D. (1959), Evaluation of tranquillizing drugs in medical out-patients: meprobamate, prochlorperazine, amobarbital sodium and placebo, *J. Amer. med. Ass.*, 171, 1649.

RINALDI, R., RUDY, L. H. AND HIMWICH, H. E. (1955), The use of frenquel in the treatment of disturbed patients with psychoses of long duration, *Amer. J. Psychiat.*, 112, 343.

ROBINSON, J. T. (1960), Discussion on an experiment with a psychiatric night hospital, *Proc. roy. Soc. Med.*, 53, 932.

ROBINSON, J. T., DAVIES, L. S. AND SACK, E. (1963), The controlled use of lysergic acid diethylamide in psychoneurosis, *J. ment. Sci.*, in press.

ROBINSON, K. (1961), *Patterns of care*, Nat. Ass. for Mental Health, London.

ROHDE, P. AND SARGANT, W. (1961), The treatment of schizophrenia in general hospitals, *Brit. med. J.*, 2, 67.

ROTHLIN, E. (1961), *Neuropsychopharmacology*, Vol. 2, Elsevier, Amsterdam.

SAMUELS, A. S. (1961), A controlled study of haloperidol: the effects of small dosages, *Amer. J. Psychiat.*, 118, 253.

SANDISON, R. A. (1954), Psychological aspects of the L.S.D. treatment of the neuroses, *J. ment. Sci.*, 100, 508.

SANDISON, R. A. (1959 a), The role of psychotropic drugs in individual therapy, *Bull. Wld. Hlth. Org.*, 21, 495.

SANDISON, R. A. (1959 b), The role of psychotropic drugs in group therapy, *Bull. Wld. Hlth. Org.*, 21, 505.

SANDISON, R. A., SPENCER, A. M. AND WHITELAW, J. D. A. (1954), The therapeutic value of lysergic acid diethylamide in mental illness, *J. ment. Sci.*, 100, 491.

SANDISON, R. A., WHITELAW, E. AND CURRIE, J. D. C. (1960), Clinical trials with Melleril in schizophrenia; a 2 year study, *J. ment. Sci.*, 106, 732.

SARGANT, W. (1958), Insulin coma for schizophrenia, *Lancet*, 2, 1370.

SARGANT, W. (1961), Drugs in the treatment of depression, *Brit. med. J.*, 1, 225.

SARGANT, W. AND DALLY, P. (1962), Treatment of anxiety states by antidepressant drugs, *Brit. med. J.*, 1, 6.

SARGANT, W. AND SHORVON, H. J. (1945), Acute war neuroses, *Arch. Neurol. Psychiat. (Chic.)*, 54, 231.

SARGANT, W. AND SLATER, E. (1954), *An introduction to physical methods of treatment in psychiatry*, 3rd ed., E. & S. Livingston, Edinburgh.

SCHOPBACH, R. R. (1961), Clinical report on methaminodiazepoxide (librium), *Amer. J. Psychiat.*, 117, 923.

SEN, G. AND BOSE, K. C. (1930), Rauwolfia serpentina: a new Indian drug for high blood pressure, *Indian med. World*, 2, 194.

SLOANE, R. B., HABIT, A. AND BATT, U. E. (1959), The use of imipramine (tofranil) for depressive states in open ward settings of a general hospital: a preliminary report, *Canad. med. Ass. J.*, 80, 540.

STANLEY, W. J. AND WALTON, D. (1961), Trifluoperazine ("stelazine"): a controlled clinical trial in chronic schizophrenia, *J. ment. Sci.*, 107, 250.

SPINELLI, D. AND PATERSON, A. S. (1962), Photographic average response indicator in electroencephalography, in preparation.

STOLL, W. A. (1949), Psychische Wirkung eines Mutterkornstoffes in ungewöhnlich schwacher Dosierung, *Schweiz. med. Wschr.*, 79, 110.

STOLLER, A. (1960), "Tofranil", a new anti-depressant drug, *Med. J. Aust.*, 1, 412.

SWANSON, D. W. AND SMITH, J. A. (1961), The use of stimulating drugs, *Amer. J. Psychiat.*, 118, 419.

TAESCHLER, M. AND SCHLAGER, E. (1961), Psychopharmaka (1) neuroleptica, *Schweiz. Apoth. Ztg.*, 99, 683.

TAESCHLER, M. AND SCHLAGER, E. (1962), Psychopharmaka (2) tranquillizer, *Schweiz. Apoth. Ztg.*, 100, 61.

THOMPSON, G. N. (1956), *Alcoholism*, C. C. Thomas, Springfield, Ill.

TIBBETTS, R. W. AND HAWKINGS, J. R. (1956), The placebo response, *J. ment. Sci.*, 102, 60.

TOBIN, J. M., BIRD, I. F. AND BOYLE, D. E. (1960), Preliminary evaluation of librium in the treatment of anxiety reactions, *Dis. nerv. Syst.*, 21, 11 (Suppl.).

TROUTON, D. S. (1957), Placebos and their psychological effects, *J. ment. Sci.*, 103, 344.

TUTEUR, W., STILLER, R. AND GLOTZER, G. (1961), *Chlorpromazine – five years later* (fifth of a series, a five years study). *Recent Advances in Biological Psychiatry*, J. WORTIS (Ed.), Vol. 3, Grune and Stratton, New York, p. 35.

UHR, L. AND MILLER, J. G. (1960), *Drugs and Behavior*, John Wiley & Sons, New York.

UNNA, K. (1943), Antagonistic effect of N-normorphine upon morphine, *J. Pharmacol. exp. Ther.*, 79, 27.

VERNIER, V. G. (1961), The pharmacology of antidepressant agents, *Dis. nerv. Syst.*, 22, no. 5, Sect. 2 – Suppl. p. 7.

VOGT, A. H. (1961), The use of stelazine and parnate in chronic, withdrawn patients, *Amer. J. Psychiat.*, 118, 256.

WALLERSTEIN, R. S. (1957), *Hospital treatment of alcoholism*, Imago, London.

WEBER, E. (1954), Ein Rauwolfia alkaloid in der Psychiatrie: seine Wirkungähnlichkeit mit Chlorpromazine, *Schweiz. med. Wschr.*, 84, 968.

WEIDMANN, H. (1961), Zur Pharmakologie psychotroper Wirkstoffe, *Schweiz. Arch. Tierheilk.*, 103, 191.

WIKLER, A. (1957), *The relation of psychiatry to pharmacology*, Williams and Wilkins, Baltimore.

WILCOX, P. H. (1951), Psychopenetration, *Dis. nerv. Syst.*, 12, 1.

WILCOX, P. H. (1961), Electrostimulation therapy and drugs, *Dis. nerv. Syst.*, 22, no. 5, Sect. 2, Suppl. p. 50.

WILLIAMS, L. (1960), *Tomorrow will be sober*, Cassell, London.

WITTS, L. J. (1959), *Medical surveys and clinical trials*, Oxford University Press.

WOLFF, P. O. (1945), The treatment of drug addicts, *Bull. Wld. Hlth. Org.*, 12, 469.

ZUKIN, F., ARNOLD, DE V. G., AND KESSLER, C. R. (1959), Comparative effects of phenaglycodol and meprobamate on anxiety reactions, *J. nerv. ment. Dis.*, 129, 193.

Subject Index

PRINTED IN THE NETHERLANDS
BY VONK & CO'S DRUKKERIJ, ZEIST